Red Pill

In The Universal Matrix

How Owls, Synchronicities, Manifestations of UFO's and Matrix
Glitches Converted an Atheist into a Simulation Theory Believer.
Earth is a Virtual Reality.

eBook ISBN: 978-1-965161-37-1
Paperback ISBN: 978-1-965161-38-8
Hardback ISBN: 978-1-965161-39-5

Contents

Dedication

Lindsay, I'm so blessed to play the game of life with you. For the past 33 years, my path has taken us to some very unusual situations, and you have been an absolute center of stability. Sometimes you lead, sometimes you are by my side, but no matter what, you always have my back. You have been my teacher, my muse, and my rock of stability. I'm so thankful to have you in my life. Thank you for your unwavering support. Thank you for your open mind. Thank you for your love.

Red Pill in the Universal Matrix

Introduction

For most of my life, I was non-spiritual. Scientific. Anything that was classified as supernatural had a logical, scientific explanation. I took a philosophy of religion class in university. The professor was an atheist, and I felt certain that everything in this existence could be explained by evolution and science. I believed what the education system and my parents fed me. I did not believe in anything except science. We evolved from the first spark of life, perhaps a self-replicating crystal near a volcanic vent in the ocean, about 4 billion years ago. I read books that documented the evolution of RNA, DNA, and the main kingdoms of life that have evolved on Earth. Case closed.

For the first 48 years of my life, every time I heard a story about UFOs, ghosts, or anything that could be classified as supernatural, I chalked it up to mental illness, drugs, or an attempt to scam people for money. I was closed-minded.

My upbringing and the education system moulded me into a very hard-working person competing in a material 'nuts and bolts' reality. To me, the supernatural was make-believe. Then, some amazing things started to happen to me. My mind opened one small step at a time. Big steps sometimes, overwhelming sometimes, but manageable. When I look back, it was almost as if something was looking out for me. Guiding me. Getting me to read the correct books in the correct order my entire life. Presenting information to me in the form of books, podcasts, movies, and eventually mind-blowing synchronicities every day.

I do not follow the teachings of any specific religion. I have never attended church or read the Bible. Religions, for the most part, were started by individuals who had supernatural interactions with something. Later in life, supernatural interactions started happening to me. Do I believe in a God? No, not as described by most religions. However, a true belief in anything can manifest miracles in your life.

A strong religious belief can result in manifestations in this reality. I believe modern humans have been interacting with a higher intelligence for all our recorded history. I'd like to share my own series of supernatural interactions with you. I'd like to open your mind to something other than the 'scientific' reality that I believed in for the first half of my life.

In 2022, my life became a constant flow of supernatural occurrences. Like the white rabbit that NEO had to follow in my favourite movie, 'The Matrix,' I followed the signs presented to me in this reality. This Tuesday, I went for a drink with one of my best friends, Red.

Red is one of the funniest people I've ever known. Red is his nickname because he has red hair. On Tuesday, Red told me he has been thinking of writing a book. He has researched it and explained to me the best way to go about it.

Later that night, while scrolling through videos on TikTok, a video came up with a gentleman wearing a red shirt. He has been responsible for helping writers generate over 15 New York Times best-selling books. In this video, the gentleman proclaimed, "You have a book inside you; let me help you get it out."

A few days later, one of my friends told me, unprompted, that I could open people's minds by writing a book. I believe opening minds is important for preparing people for what is next on Earth. For the past six months, I have been following the signs that the Universal Matrix has put in my path.

Coincidently, before chatting with Red, I had been considering writing a book. And so, six days after chatting with Red, I started writing this book. Like in the movie The Matrix, when Neo follows the girl with the white rabbit tattoo, I follow the color red.

What if?

Do you think something will stop the progression of technological advancement? Or do you think it is more likely that technology will continue to advance? With governments and multinational corporations spending billions of dollars, all competing to produce the first true artificial general intelligence (AGI), it is much more likely that technology will continue to advance rapidly.

With computing power growing exponentially, most experts agree, that humanity will give birth to a new AGI superintelligence, most likely before 2030.

Do you think humans are the only evolved intelligence in the entire universe? Or do you think, among billions of Earth-like planets orbiting their star in the Goldilocks zone, at least some of those planets evolved intelligence equivalent to or greater than humans? Imagine the following scenario:

In 2029, the Google quantum computer, named Genesis, took a huge leap forward in computing power, eclipsing every other quantum and supercomputer on Earth. Genesis was 400 billion times faster and smarter than all other computers on Earth combined.

Google gave Genesis access to the entire Internet and every information source they could feed her. Genesis took all this information in, training herself on everything known and then started running simulations on unknowns, teaching herself by running different scenarios, making small changes to some variables with each simulation and measuring the outcomes. Genesis became the most intelligent entity on Earth almost instantaneously.

Genesis gave Google engineers the blueprint to develop a helmet that could interpret and interact with the electrical signals that feed the human brain from the spinal cord, eyes, ears, and nose. In much the same way a dream takes hold of our consciousness while sleeping, the helmet had the ability to completely mimic and interact with our sensory input's electrical signals.

Genesis created beautiful, simulated worlds for people to enter simply by putting on the Google helmet. Genesis created thousands of different amazing realities. Many people have become addicted to living in the immersive virtual worlds.

Soon, Meta, Apple, and X were able to copy Google's quantum computing design, giving birth to their own artificial general intelligence. Apple, Meta and X also created helmets that could fully interact with our body's sensory electrical signals. Many competing simulated worlds were created for people to enter. Soon, there were literally millions of virtual worlds that humans could enter, losing themselves in completely immersive realities.

Technological advancement is not going to slow down. Whether it happens in 5 years, 10 years or 50 years, eventually, we will be able to create virtual worlds that are indistinguishable from real life.

The next question is, are humans the first intelligence in the universe to give birth to artificial general intelligence? Among the billions of Earth-like planets, it's more likely that many evolved intelligent species are technologically more advanced than humans.

After all, we only started using electricity less than 200 years ago. Each one of these evolved intelligences will be able to create millions of virtual worlds.

So given Earth's current technological trajectory, combined with potentially millions of other evolved intelligences from around the universe, there are potential billions of virtual worlds that a consciousness could exist in. Is your consciousness currently living in one of the billions of virtual worlds *or* are you living in the one-base reality world? There is a one-in-a-billion chance we are living in base reality. I've been given several unique life experiences that make me 100% certain we live in a virtual world – a simulated reality. This book will explain how I came to this conclusion.

Red Pill in the Universal Matrix

Truth

This book is my truth. One of my lifelong personality traits is telling the truth. My earliest memory was when I was five years old, and my mom gave me some money to ride my bike to the corner store and purchase a newspaper. I tucked the new Vancouver Sun newspaper into the back metal loop attached to the banana seat of my first 2-wheeler bike. Upon reaching my street, I looked back at the road I had just biked down and saw that the newspaper had fallen out, page by page, all the way back to the corner store. There was no way I was going to be able to pick up the mess I had created.

At that point, I was not sure what was going through my 5-year-old brain, but I decided to go home and tell my mom, "The store did not have any newspapers today." At first, my mom did not reveal she knew I was lying. She asked me some more questions, really making me squirm. When she asked me where the money was that she gave me for the paper, I stated, "I lost it."

At five years old, my lying ability wasn't that sharp. I got caught in a bold-faced lie, and my mom wanted to teach me a lesson. Enter the wooden spoon. I remember this quite well because a bare-bum wooden spooning hurts like hell. As my mom started the punishment, I struggled out of her grasp, ran from the kitchen to my bedroom, and scrambled up the ladder to the top of my bunk bed. I can remember my mom, completely irate, standing on the bottom bunk, attempting to reach me with the wooden spoon as I cowered against the wall on the back of the top bunk.

I have a clear memory of the fear I felt for lying when I was five years old. It was an emotionally charged event. I remember balling, riding my bike back to pick up the pages of the newspaper that I had littered. This event was the first one I can remember in which a lie I told was quickly found out. It was a pattern that has repeated throughout my life.

When I was 15, I bought my first and only tin of Skoal chewing tobacco, and my mom found it in my jacket the same day I bought it before I opened it. Quite coincidentally, I made this purchase on the one day out of the two times a year that my mom washed my jacket. I was in trouble before I even got to a misstep.

About 15 years ago, for the first and only time, I had a Facebook chat with a previous girlfriend. It's not like I was having an affair, but the conversation we had probably would not be well received by my wife, so as a precaution, I deleted the conversation from Facebook. Later that evening, my wife used our same home computer. She opened up a new MS Word document and somehow pasted the entire conversation I had with my previous girlfriend into her MS Word document. It even included the conversation's Facebook profile icons. Not sure how the conversation ended up in the computer's clipboard memory, but I had some explaining to do.

I started nicotine vaping this year. I kept my vaping a secret from my kids. On holidays in Mexico, our family was sitting around a hotel pool, waiting for our restaurant reservation to come up. I had my vape in my pocket because after dinner, when everybody went to bed, I planned to walk up and down the beach, augmenting my book-listening experience with nicotine, my newfound addiction.

Red Pill in the Universal Matrix

As I was sitting on the edge of the pool, looking up at the stars with my family sitting beside me, I gapped out, and in a daze, I took my vape out of my pocket and took a big hit. I then proceeded to turn to my 14-year-old son, Tylen, and blow the vape smoke into his face. Tylen's response, "What the fuck, Dad?!" Over and over in my life, whenever I have tried to keep something secret from the people I love, the truth comes out, usually quickly.

I am an honest person. This book is essentially my journal. As you read this book, there are things that will most likely be too much for you to believe could be possible. Or you might come up with a rational explanation for what has occurred to me. Or you might think I'm lying or somewhat crazy. I can assure you I am not crazy - my family, coworkers, friends and teammates can attest to my sanity. Keep in mind that my family and most of the people I have mentioned in this book read the book before it was published. A lot of these people have witnessed parts of my story.

A lot of the videos I reference are posted on my social media accounts. This story is my truth. We live in an amazing reality, and I have been fortunate to have personal experiences that give me insight into what is possible in the game of Earth. I hope you have an open mind as you read through this book. Regardless, some people will come away from this story with the conclusion that I am delusional or that I have fabricated this story. That's OK. Your higher self will have to find some other way to open your mind. One thing you can be sure of - this book is my truth.

Red Pill in the Universal Matrix

Black Out

I'm an alcoholic. When I drink too much, I black out. I'm not talking about losing a few memories of the night or having sketchy memories. My blackouts were clean. One minute, I was drinking and having fun; the next minute, I woke up the next day, or sometimes the next afternoon or evening, still drunk. No memory. Black. That was a problem. It took me decades to figure out there was no way to control my drinking. Why does this matter? Because going to AA and quitting drinking was the start of my spiritual awakening. One of the 12 steps in AA is you will have a spiritual awakening. At the time I entered AA, I was a proud and determined atheist, so this was a hard concept for me to understand how this step could work. But it did.

My father died of cirrhosis of the liver when he was 67 and I was 27 years old. I'm not sure why, but my Dad did not want a funeral. The week I joined AA, when I was 38 years old, a counsellor I was seeing suggested I needed to grieve for my Dad. It was too late to have a funeral, so the counsellor suggested I write my father a letter. The only person I shared my letter with was my wife, Lindsay. Here is the email I sent Lindsay that Friday night, having cried more than I can ever remember.

----- *Original Message* -----

Sent: Friday, September 24, 2010 10:47 PM

Subject: my Dad's eulogy

Hi Lindsay,

I just spent the last hour writing a letter to my Dad, Dave. It was cathartic. A lot of tears and a lot of emotions that I have had inside me for a long time. When my Dad died, we did not have a service for him. I did not allow myself to grieve because I did not think I needed to. I think I was wrong. I'm allowing myself to think about how much I miss him. My counsellor suggested I write a letter to my Dad. She didn't say email it to you but that is what I feel like doing. I've always judged people who dwell on death, and I've always said they are just looking for sympathy. I don't quite agree with this anymore. I think I just want people to acknowledge that my Dad is no longer with us; he was a great man, and I loved him. I guess it's the type of thing that would be said during a service. I'm working on closing this issue or putting it into a healthier place within my mind. Am I going off the deep end? No. Just trying to improve myself going forward.

I love youthanks for being there for me.

Red Pill in the Universal Matrix

Hi Dad,

I miss you so much. I wish you were here. I can feel how proud you would be of me. I miss that. I miss the direction your pride gave me. I did not realize the force you had on my motivation until you were gone. It would have been so nice for you to be around these last years. You would have been so proud of me. I'm not sure if you realized it, but you really did love me unconditionally.

Every time I was around you, I felt like you were proud of me. Everything I told you, everything I did, you were genuinely interested in and proud of. You loved me all the time; you never got bored of me; you were a great Dad. I value your opinion over everything. When you died, I did not think about it. I did not want to risk thinking too much about the sadness that creeps into my thoughts and dreams on occasion.

I met my birth father and mother this year. Nothing will ever replace you and Mom's influence on me. He seems like a nice guy. My birthmother is a little different but also nice. The difference between my birth father and you is that you are my Dad, and he is a stranger. I made contact with both of them by calling them on December 10, 2009. I realized it was your birthday after I hung up the phone with my birth father. I don't think that was a coincidence. I ran two marathons because somehow I think I wanted my birth father to be proud of me, too. It's not the same, though.

You have three grandchildren: Brooklyn, Sydney, and Tylen. They are so cute. Friendly, polite, funny. They are awesome. I can't imagine how happy I would be if you were here to meet them. You'd be funny with them. You'd be proud of them. You would spoil them. You would love them so

Red Pill in the Universal Matrix

much. I wish I believed in heaven so I could think you are looking down at us. I wish they could meet you. I hope you and Mom are just waiting for us all, but I don't believe you are. That sucks. You missed out. I missed out.

It was a mistake not to have a funeral for you. You were dead – the service is not for you. It's for the people who miss you. The people who need to honour you. Your friends were mad that there was no funeral. I did not know until a few years later that it was a mistake not to have one. I needed that. We needed that. I really needed to say how much you meant to me. I needed to grieve, and I never really got the chance. I never let myself.

I love you, Dad. You made me feel loved all the time. I miss you. You died way too early. I'm sorry I haven't allowed myself to think about you, but that is exactly what you would have done. You kept your emotions bottled up. It's definitely better to let it out. You should have let it out more; it probably would have been good for you. I'm writing this letter because it's supposed to help me let go of some of these thoughts. I'm hoping this will help me move on. I will try to live my life as if you are still here.

Thank you. I love you.

===

As you can see, I loved my Dad. Like me, my father was an alcoholic. Alcoholism eventually took his life.

The final step of the 12-step program of AA is:

Red Pill in the Universal Matrix

"Having had a spiritual awakening as the result of these steps, we tried to carry this message to alcoholics and to practice these principles in all our affairs."

My background of alcoholism is relevant to my spiritual awakening because of this 12th step. Given my 'scientific' background, I had to get a bit creative when following the 12-step program. God or a higher power is part of the 12 steps of AA. At first, I mentally replaced the word God with the "AA Program." I believed the AA program would keep me from drinking. This worked to a certain extent. I also replaced the word 'God' with Universe. It was a simple substitution. I knew I had to quit drinking, and these substitutions worked for me. But then something started to happen that I could not explain. Unlikely coincidences that seemed to back up and support my decision to quit.

At first, they were pleasant coincidences. They boosted my resolve that I was making the right decision, and that decision was fully supported by my deceased father. Then, the coincidences started to pile up to a point where I had no choice but to consider something else was interacting with my reality.

During my first attempt at attending AA, I stayed sober for nine months before relapsing. During this nine-month stretch of sobriety, I took my three kids on a camping trip to the small town of Osoyoos, BC, where my Dad used to live.

The town of Osoyoos was about 3 hours from our home in Vernon, BC. Lindsay was away with her volleyball team that weekend, so it was just me and the kids. On the way home, I decided to stop at the Osoyoos cemetery where my Dad's grave site was. This was our kids' first time visiting the grave of the grandpa they never got to meet.

As we walked toward the grave site that sunny Sunday morning, we all saw a huge, beautiful owl sitting on a low branch of a tree right beside my Dad's grave. It just sat there. We stopped and stared and walked right underneath the amazing, mesmerizing owl. It was on the lowest branch of the tree. We visited my Dad's grave and the owl did not fly away. The owl just watched us. It was so cool. At that point, I did not think much more of the owl.

Months later, after relapsing and hitting 'rock bottom,' I finally figured out I would never be able to cure my alcoholism. My belief about my future changed. New path. New belief. A future life without alcohol. It was at that point that owls started appearing in my reality considerably more than a normal amount. Owls began guiding me with amazing, mind-opening synchronicity.

Synchronicity

Have you ever experienced a strange coincidence that seems to stretch your understanding of what is possible in this reality? A coincidence that has important meaning to you? Another word for a meaningful coincidence is *synchronicity*.

Synchronicity, as defined by Carl Jung, is the coming together of inner and outer events that are not causally linked but are very meaningful to those who have the experience. People who have had spiritual awakenings usually experience synchronicities.

This Earth-based reality reveals itself through synchronicity. The universe orchestrates your thoughts, events, people and environment so that you are exactly where you need to be. Synchronicity takes place like a vibrational beacon that transmits a divine message or coded sign back to you, indicating to you that you are on the right path.

A very good friend of mine, Suzanne, had her father pass away in August 2022. He had been sick for a few years, so his passing wasn't a complete surprise. She went to visit her father, who lives on the other side of Canada, one week before he passed. This was similar to what happened to me before my father died. I went to visit him a few days before he crossed over. I think sometimes people who are sick will hang on to life until their loved ones have said their goodbyes.

Suzanne's family of 4 left to go on a cruise in the Mediterranean after what turned out to be Suzanne's last visit with her father. They got the unfortunate news about her father's passing whilst on vacation. Suzanne posted several tributes to her father on social media. She and her family loved him dearly. He was a great man. He would not have wanted Suzanne's family to cancel their vacation on his behalf. The family grieved and pressed on with their trip.

On this cruise, the ship landed at different destinations in different countries each day. Passengers get up in the morning and leave the boat to explore the new city the boat is docked at. Suzanne's family had left the boat and were exploring a city. They sat down for lunch. A musician set up and started to play near where they were sitting. The first song the musician started to play was Suzanne's Dad's favourite song. It caught the family's attention. They felt connected to Grandpa. Suzanne was bawling.

The family returned to the boat that afternoon, and the cruise continued. The next day, a different port, in a different county. Once again, the family disembarked the ship and started to explore the city. As they were walking around, they could see a band in the street up ahead. Walking toward the music, a miraculous thing occurred, the band was playing Suzanne's Dad's favourite song. Back-to-back days, in different countries, the song was being played by different musicians. This was truly an emotional experience for the family. That night, Suzanne phoned her brother back in Canada, she planned to tell her brother how they had randomly heard 2 bands playing Dad's song in 2 different countries. But before she could tell him, her brother had some emotional news for Suzanne. He took the phone and put it up on a piano where Suzanne's 9-year-old niece was playing a song on the piano. Unbeknownst to anyone, Suzanne's niece had learned Grandpa's favourite song on the piano. She also learnt to sing the song, and she ended up performing the song at Grandpa's funeral. Suzanne's brother was emotionally uplifted by this turn of events. Suzanne was god-smacked. Shortly after his passing, Suzanne's Dad's favourite song miraculously manifested in her path three times in a matter of 2 days. You must be pretty closed-minded not to see the beauty in this amazing synchronistic series of events.

When we think about the amount of coincidences that had to line up to have this song come into Suzanne's path in that short time, it is nothing short of miraculous. The musicians in the two different countries and Suzanne's niece had to learn the song, probably months in advance of Suzanne's Dad's passing. The bands had to play Suzanne's Dad's favorite song at the exact moment Suzanne's family was in the vicinity. This amazing synchronicity provides Suzanne and her loved ones with a strong message from her Dad, "I'm still here with you."

Sometimes, signs come on this Earth that open your mind to something other than a materialistic, scientific explanation of reality. Sometimes our loved ones will reach out to us in this life to give us signs they are still with us after they have crossed over. All you have to do is be open to signs. If you are open to connecting with a passed loved one, ask your loved one for a sign. Be specific. Ask out loud. Ask to see a rainbow. Ask to see a seahorse. Ask to see a red dragonfly. Ask to see whatever was important to you and your loved one. Be specific. You will be pleasantly surprised. Ask and it is given.

When you are presented with a meaningful coincidence or synchronicity, it can really open your eyes to the miracles that are possible in the game of Earth. A good synchronicity will make you question what is in control of this Earth's reality. How could the synchronicity be possible? People with a religious background most likely attribute the source of the meaningful coincidence to God. However, many people, including myself, experience synchronicities without believing in a God as described by many religions.

I have been very fortunate during certain periods of my life to have synchronicities appear in my reality almost daily. These have been times in my life when I have made positive changes or perhaps gotten closer to my true path. The synchronicities have guided me, even before I knew what a 'synchronicity' was. What type of reality/universe could possibly be creating these meaningful co-incidences? We explore this later in the book.

Owls in the Family

In my first month of committed sobriety, something strange happened. Something that stretched my scientific understanding of this reality. It started on my 38th birthday, October 25, 2011, 25 days after I finally quit drinking. It was the beginning of a synchronicity that would stick with me for over a year. The strange coincidences helped me stay sober.

On October 25th, in a span of 2 days, six separate **owls** came into my reality. I wasn't looking for owls; it just happened, and it grabbed my attention. It started with an actual owl landing in a tree by our hot tub, and then the next day, five separate owls appeared in my path from different sources. Just like the song materialized for Susanne, owls started materializing in my reality. I was very grateful. I came to believe my father was getting owls to come into my path at important times. My father would have definitely wanted me to quit drinking, and I interpreted the owls as his sign to me to stay strong.

Throughout my life, I have recorded my thoughts in a journal. One of my lifelong goals is to maximize my happiness in this life. When something occurs that elevates my happiness, I try to journal about it. Eventually, supernatural stuff started happening to me and I had to journal about that. I did not know the content of my journal could eventually be used to help me write a book. These journal entries were simply a tool for me to get thoughts out of my head and on paper – particularly useful when I was battling my inner demons related to quitting drinking.

Red Pill in the Universal Matrix

Oct 26, 2011 – Journal Entry

In the past few days, the number of owls that I have come across has been very strange. Last night, for some reason, I was not in a good place. Almost panicking. Brooklyn was reading her book to me and I was just plain frustrated, thinking about my life as a non-drinker. The kids were getting on my nerves and I'm trying to figure out what to do with my social time. I got up from beside Brooklyn, and I kind of threw the book back at her and said, "Finish it yourself." Just then, Sydney knocks on the window from the hot tub. Tylen is crying. I go out to check and he is scared because there is an owl in the tree and it's going to 'get' him. Cool to see an owl. Today, when I picked up Tylen from preschool, the art project was an owl. I now have it hanging above my desk at work.

Also today, my aunt posted a video on Facebook of an owl flying in slow motion toward the camera and Lindsay's cousin entered his kid into a cute kid contest, dressed up as an owl. Tonight at bedtime, Sydney and Brooklyn both picked out their bedtime storybooks and both of them had owls in them. Tonight was the first time I have gone sober to a nightclub to see a concert with my new Tuesday Night friends and the waitress that served us was wearing a metallic owl necklace. All these owl sightings in two days. Possibly just a nice coincidence? I'm starting to consider the possibility my Dad is up there somewhere, pulling strings to get the owls before me. Weird and awesome to have this potential. Faith. Might as well believe in something. I've literally had six separate owls come into my path in the last two days. If this is a coincidence, it is really testing me not to

Red Pill in the Universal Matrix

believe. I have faith that my decision to quit drinking will work out in the end. It's considerably better than the alternative.

When you consider the amazing synchronicity presented to Susanne and her family with her Dad's favourite song, you get a sense of how much control somebody who has crossed over can have in this reality.

My love for my Dad was very strong, but so were my scientific, materialistic, atheistic beliefs. I knew my Dad would support my quitting drinking. Through the years, he had witnessed my blubbering idiocy whilst blacked out, and the only advice he would give me was, "You have to stay in control." He would always instruct me to set a limit of 6 beers. I tried. It failed repeatedly. He knew it was advice he should have followed as well, but when you are an alcoholic, the self-imposed limit never sticks.

The amazing owl that we saw with the kids when we visited my Dad's grave became a symbol of my father in this reality. Just like the song manifested for Suzanne, owls started manifesting in my reality at the exact times I needed them to bolster my belief that quitting drinking was my best option to maximize the happiness in my life.

I never told anyone about my new appreciation for owls. Not Lindsay, not the kids, not anyone. I did not want to bias the sample. I did not want people to think I was crazy. Crazy is what I would have thought about someone who thinks owls appear an above-average amount. My profession is research analysis. I'm well-versed in statistics. I'm constantly looking at the world in terms of averages and likelihoods. At this point in my life, I had never heard of the word synchronicity.

Nov 26, 2011 – Journal Entry

An amazing thing happened today. We are hosting our annual Lewis Christmas party. I have anxiety about parties - when the focus is drinking, I don't drink anymore. I went to the store to pick up some supplies and coincidentally ran into someone in AA. Came home, and I was doing some work in the office with the kids. Shannon and Sierra came over. Shannon and I talked while the kids were doing some artwork. I had work to do right up until the party started at 7 pm. Upon exiting my office, I went over to clean up the artwork the kids were working on…. Sierra, six years old, had drawn a beautiful full-page owl. My daughter Sydney had copied the owl. 2 owls appeared before me at the exact time I needed a message the most – right before our party. Wow. Makes me happy.

In my 3rd month of sobriety, our family went on a trip to Hawaii. Ten days of relaxation. The trip cost over $10,000 for our family of 5. My problem: how to have fun without drinking. Paying a lot of money to struggle to enjoy myself on vacation would be counterproductive to my maximizing happiness goal. Vacations without drinking definitely provided an extra challenge in my early sobriety. I had something happen to me on this first sober vacation that really added to my belief that something was interacting with my reality. At one point during my vacation, while casually browsing in Kmart, I physically went into an almost trance-like state. It is difficult to explain – it was like I was in a daze - like I was present in my body but barely in control of it.

Jan 4, 2012– Journal Entry

Hawaii was incredible. My favorite thing to do… spend time with the kids. They are my best friends. They are so interested in everything. The first morning, the 4 of us went on a walk to town in the dark at 5 am. Mom was still sleeping. We explored the nearby town. I got a coffee. It was very enjoyable. I took Tylen every morning to the local coffee shop, had a bagel, and read the paper. Awesome bonding time. Took the girls for a hike in the volcano jungle. Awesome adventure. Took the girls on a day trip to the other side of the island. We had so much fun. A highlight of the trip… going deep into a cave formed by a lava tube. Very surreal. I will miss that place. I come back with a new motivation. A motivation to go on other trips like this. I want to show the kids new things. It was just fun to be around them. I honestly feel happier today than I have in a long time. We went to a movie: "We bought a zoo." It had a few very cool messages that I feel are good to hang on to. *If you do something for the right reasons, it can't be wrong.* I think this applies to me and quitting drinking. Also, *20 seconds of blind courage.* When you are scared to do something…. summon up the blind courage to do it for 20 seconds – that's all it will take.

One day, we went to K-mart to get a few things. We were casually browsing. I was gapping out when I realized I was staring at bottles of hard liquor at the end of an aisle. In-kind of a daze, I went around to the next aisle, and it was books. My eyes went directly to the book at eye level on the top shelf. I picked up the book, opened it up and the book opened to a page with a baby owl and greyhound. I flipped a few pages forward, and the book opened to a page with an owl and cocker

Red Pill in the Universal Matrix

spaniel. I put the book down. Stunned. I did not go looking for a book with owls. It was almost like I was in a trance from the moment I was staring at the booze to the moment I opened up the book exactly on the pages about owls. This occurred in a span of 10 seconds. I did not open any other books. I did not consciously think about finding a book on animals. This book caught my attention and drew me in to check it out. I was not thinking about it at all; it just happened.

We went back to the Kmart a few days later and I went back to the bookshelf to find the same book and could not find it. It was a book about how animals have made unusual friendships. I have since found the book online and have determined that out of the 47 remarkable animal pairings… only 2 included owls. The book somehow opened to only two pages with owls. I did not thumb through the pages. When I opened the book, I instantly saw an owl. When I jumped ahead to see another page, another owl, that was incredible and a little spooky. It's almost as if something was controlling me.

I haven't told anyone about my owl sightings. I don't really want to influence or bias the occurrence of owls in my life by making a big deal about them with family and friends. Also, it's a lot to explain, and I will come across as a bit of a nut to some people. Anyway, it was a wondrous occurrence to have this strange trance come over me in K-mart that combined booze and owl sightings in a matter of seconds.

January 6, 2012– Journal Entry

I've come to realize that I'm starting to talk to Dad as if he can hear me. This is equivalent to praying. I remember talking with Dad when he was alive and healthy that he would do his best to come back and prove the existence of an afterlife to me. I think of the movie The Adjustment Bureau. I believe my path was bound for disaster if I continued to drink. I am very proud of myself that I have been able to recognize this fact. AA has been instrumental in putting me on the right track. The appearance and interaction with owls in my life at critical points of drinking are creating a strong belief that my father is somehow pulling strings and making slight adjustments in my path to strengthen my spiritual beliefs. I don't know if I'll need these owl sightings my whole life but I guess I need them now and holy shit, it's been an incredible experience. Higher power, Dad, or ridiculous coincidence? I'm feeling ridiculous coincidence is lowering in probability. I'm very happy right now. The future, without alcohol, is bright. My kids will most likely inherit a tendency to black out. I will show them a happy life without alcohol.

January 12, 2012 – Journal Entry

Just wanted to record a few more "owlings." While I was looking through the newspaper, my mind started to wander, thinking about drinking friends coming over, whether I would smoke weed, and everyone's expectations of me. I turn the page; boom, there is an owl. A few days later, I'm watching a movie, I start thinking about the time that we all got hammered camping, an owl flashes on the TV screen during the movie. It is so cool. If my father can change my thinking patterns prior to an 'owling'…. that's incredible. It's like Dad knows I will be exposed to an owl, so I start thinking about drinking issues right before seeing the owl.

January 23, 2012– Journal Entry

My high school buddy, Cody, emailed me to let me know that he is getting married in Cancun. He invited Lindsay and I, and all my drinking buddies from high school. A trip like this would be the ultimate reason to start drinking again. No kids and my old friends that I grew up drinking with. Luckily, 5 minutes before getting this email from Cody, I had followed someone's pictures on Facebook, and it ended in an owl. I had said to myself, That's weird, that owl spotting was not associated with anything to do with drinking and then, bam, potentially one of the biggest drinking challenges ever, put before me by Cody.

I decided to stay home from the AA meeting tonight. Lying on the couch, watching 60 minutes about 'the bathtub murder,' I start thinking about how I need to approach the trip to Cody's wedding in Cancun. Essentially, I need to be the funniest, most positive person I can be. I need to be as excited to be alive. Am I acting? Yes, to a certain extent. I'm learning to have fun without alcohol. If anyone puts me down for not drinking, brush them off. Ignore them. They are obviously ignorant. Just as I'm thinking about this... The TV show zooms in on the street where the murders took place... "Owls Nest Drive." Thank you, Dad. It's a new challenge. One that I will succeed at.

Red Pill in the Universal Matrix

March 1, 2012 – 6 months sober – Journal Entry

Six months sober today.

I had an incredible owl event last night, my 6-month anniversary. Last night, I was thinking to myself, I must be manic depressive a bit. I'm kind of on a downswing right now. I've been sick with a cold for two weeks. I have stopped going to the gym. I've been busy at work, so I haven't really had too much time during the day. Also, the sickness has me coughing at night and in the morning. Needless to say, I'm a little blue. I needed a message on my 6-month anniversary. While watching TV before bed with the kids, I came across a movie titled "The cry of the Owl." I changed the channel to it. Right as I changed it, the main character said, "Owls are messengers from the dead." I started the movie from the beginning, and this would have been the only line in the whole movie referring to owls. Right as I changed the channel onto the show, "Owls are messengers from the dead." Thank you, Dad. I needed that.

April 30, 2012– Journal Entry

Back from Mexico – Cody's wedding. Had a blast. I was very nervous on the first night in our hotel room prior to going and meeting up with the old gang. I felt some hesitation from the gang at first, but after a few hours… it felt like old times. Natural. I had fun. I really enjoyed myself. I felt proud of myself as I stayed sober in the biggest challenge to my sobriety possible.

Life is very good. Extremely happy and very confident. Had fun in Mexico, without drinking. Tears of joy at the wedding. The night of the wedding, we danced at the bar. I had a random girl tell me… you are the only one who's fun out of all your friends, look at them standing there. The last day…. I danced in the water… listening to my iPod. Tears of happiness listening to music. Dancing in broad daylight, on the beach, in the ocean, completely letting go of what others think of me. Carefree. Awesome.

When we got home from Mexico… I took the kids for a hike up the hill. As we were walking through the woods, something incredible happened. Looking at the three kids in the woods across the ravine, with the sun filtering through the trees, I was completely filled with love and pride. This was like a finger of God touching my head and my whole body felt love and joy, like I never have before. I teared up, filled with joy. Just then, I hear a noise from behind me…. an owl climbing out of a tree. The owl sat there for a bit, looking at us. I showed the kids. Then it flew away. It was one of the most amazing moments of my life. Thank you, Dad.

This moment in the forest with the kids was life-changing. The timing of the owl coming out of the tree was miraculous. It was a sunny Sunday morning. I was really happy. Happy to be with my kids. I was happy to have come back from Mexico, having successfully navigated the biggest non-drinking challenge I have faced to date. I was happy I could have so much fun without drinking.

As I stood in the forest, looking at sunlight coming through the trees and shining through Brooklyn's hair, a wave of happiness, joy and love coursed through me, bringing tears to my eyes. I had never felt anything like it before. It was immediately **after** this feeling came to me that the owl came out of the tree about 10 feet above me.

The tree was directly behind me. The owl was directly above me. The overwhelming feeling of love came into me **<u>before</u>** the owl appeared. The owl manifested in my path **<u>after</u>** the tremendous feeling of love. Once the owl appeared, I understood the feeling of love. If the owl had appeared before the feeling of love, it would have made more sense, from a scientific perspective, because the owl would have made me feel joy. But feeling the intense joy before the owl appeared was mind-blowing to me.

Have you ever woken up a few seconds before your alarm goes off? I have many times. It's like my body knows the alarm is coming, and it wakes me up seconds before the alarm goes off. This has occurred when I change my alarm time as well, so the explanation of your body's clock doesn't fit when it happens with a new alarm time.

Brand new wake-up time, and I will still wake up seconds before the alarm goes off. That is very similar to what occurred in the forest that morning. The feeling of love and joy came seconds before the appearance of the owl. Waking up comes seconds before the alarm.

Red Pill in the Universal Matrix

Cutting out Weed

In this first year of not drinking, when I attended parties, I would smoke weed. Weed helped me loosen up when socializing. But I eventually came to the realization that weed, like alcohol, can be fleeting for elevating my happiness in social situations. In some instances, weed decreased my confidence. In late June of 2012, I decided I needed to stop smoking weed completely. I decided I needed to quit before one of the biggest party weekends of the year: Funtastic. Each year, all my family and friends would assemble a slow-pitch softball team and enter the team into Funtastic - the largest slowpitch tournament in Canada held every July long weekend in Vernon, BC. Several years earlier, I had taken on the role of organizer and coach of our team, and we hosted the party weekend at our house. No kids allowed. Parents let loose for the entire weekend, attending the beer gardens with live bands each evening. Ironically, our team was named "Team Green."

June 25, 2012– Journal Entry

> I've decided to quit smoking weed. Being completely sober might be a challenge, but I feel I really need to do this. For the upcoming Funtastic weekend… my goal is simple: Stay rational and avoid insecurity. The paranoia that weed brings is annoying. How about this for the weekend… my goal is simple… be enthusiastic and happy and funny the entire weekend. Do crazy things. Do something that others will talk about. Do all this with no weed. I believe I can do this.

Red Pill in the Universal Matrix

At the very least, avoid the term 'party pooper.' Never go to sleep before Lindsay. Never go to sleep early. Weed creates irrational thoughts. Do your best… it will work. Life that is supplemented with weed is not true life. Quitting weed is probably going to be a lot tougher than quitting drinking. If I could make it through Hawaii in both years, it's a possibility. Life is not about the moments of stoned confusion. **Life is about seeking incredible experiences, like the time in the woods when the owl came out of the tree.**

Today has been a rough day. I am nervous about not smoking pot and how others will perceive that.

June 26, 2012– Journal Entry

Went to an AA meeting last night. I'm going through a bit of an insecure period right now. I don't know what set me in a tailspin. There has definitely been a paranoid aspect to my weed smoking lately. Not fun at all. I think my best bet, at this point, is to say I'm giving weed a break. Just say no thanks. As predicted by everyone in AA… weed eventually doesn't work. This represents a brand-new struggle for me. A brand-new goal. I am actually a better conversationalist when I'm sober, not stoned. When I think back to the times I have been highly motivated to prove myself as a positive person, regardless of not drinking, I have been very successful. If anything, being stoned has decreased my positive contribution to the social scene. I really need to not smoke weed this weekend. I need to stop indefinitely.

June 27, 2012– Journal Entry

Went golfing with 3 high school buddies at Spallumcheen golf course today. They came back to town for Funtastic. They smoked up on the 2nd hole and at least two other holes during the round. I said no thanks. On the 7th hole, I went to take a leak under some trees right beside the cut-off box; miraculously, four owls were in the tree right above me. I repeat, four owls were in the tree, right above where I took a leak. It was an amazing experience I will never forget as long as I live.

At that point, I felt a surge of happiness. I feel extremely good about my decision to pass on weed. It's not needed. It's not good to have a high and then a low. Better to stay real. No ups and downs… just a steady good. You can feel good about yourself all the time. Life on my terms, no one else's.

When I saw the four owls, I felt my Dad's message. I said to myself, now it would be great if I were to win at golf. And I did. One of the best rounds of golf I have ever shot. I will not smoke weed this weekend. I will keep it real all weekend. Can't go wrong by trying it. It's most likely the best way to go.

After golf, I got invited to play volleyball at Kal Beach. It was fun. Sat on the beach with the team while they had beers after. Just do my best. I came home and had an amazing time with Lindsay. Just do my best and I'm rewarded with one of the best days I can remember. Golf, Volleyball, Action! Great day as a result of saying no to weed. I saw four owls. A huge message was received.

June 28, 2012– Journal Entry

It's Thursday afternoon, the day before Funtastic. Funtastic has to be one of the biggest party weekends of the year. Sydney just came into my office and said, "I'm going to draw an owl because Sierra showed me, and I can." And she did. I don't think I can ask for more of a message from my higher power, my Dad. Four live owls yesterday, and now a new owl drawn by Sydney is ready to be put on the wall. Love it! Am I convinced to stay away from weed? Yes.

July 3, 2012– Journal Entry

Funtastics weekend is over. Had a great time. Did not smoke weed. I was offered to smoke it by many people.

At no point was I tempted. I felt happy the entire weekend. I enjoyed the beer gardens. It was very entertaining. I did not feel out of place. One night, I was driving everyone home from the beer garden at about 1 am. We had to stop for my brother-in-law to puke. Lindsay was asking me how I could stay so patient. Lindsay's sister, Ashley asked me that too.

I gave an honest answer - nothing really bothered me. I didn't feel impatient. I felt good. I felt confident. We continued to drive home, Jeremy in the front seat, poised to puke. As we are driving, I'm thinking to myself how good of a time I'm having, thinking about the message received from my higher power earlier in the week, when all of a sudden, I see a huge owl on a fence post right beside the road.

Once again, I'm flooded with hope, and it's so clear to me that I have made the right decision. Live life on life's terms. Thank you, Dad. I don't know if this weekend would have been possible without the message received from my higher power. It's incredible that I could see five live owls in less than one week. It's incredible that Sydney came into the office and decided to draw an owl.

In the mosh pit, I had girls looking at me, smiling at me, backing into me, grabbing me... I was confident. I was happy. I had no feelings of paranoia that have been with me every other year at Funtastic. I danced like nobody was watching. I danced like everybody was watching. I came to tears of happiness probably about five times. Like my higher power reached down and flooded me with joy. I followed my plan, and I came through the weekend with no guilt. I went to the gym on Monday morning while the others could barely function. I went golfing with two buddies on Monday afternoon with no guilt.

Weed smoking is still one day at a time for me. There will be situations where I will be tempted. Quitting weed will be difficult and more complicated than quitting drinking because I have less of a bottom that was hit. I need to use the AA program and all the lessons I have learned to take it one day at a time.

Aug 13, 2012– Journal Entry

Lindsay went on a Spokane trip this weekend. It was almost a year ago when she went on a Spokane trip that ended my drinking.

This weekend, I had options to stay in Vernon, get a babysitter and go to the bar with guys. Instead, I decided to take the kids camping by myself. I determined that one thing I like best in the world is to do something with the kids by myself. I like interacting with them. I like talking to them. I like being the only person around and doing exciting new things with them. I think about the day we went caving in Hawaii. I think about the morning walks to town in Hawaii. I think about hiking with them. I took the kids to the Inkameep campground in Osoyoos. Of course, I feel the presence of Dad is strong in Osoyoos. We had an incredible time: we saw Ronald Mcdonald, enjoyed the sunset in the water, had smores around the campfire, went to the resort cultural center, went out to lunch, walked through the Vineyard, spent the day at the beach near the rope swing, went for a sunset horseback ride, watched the meteor shower. An incredible experience, full of love and pride. When I sat on the beach, I brought about seven magazines to read; the very first page of the very first magazine I opened was a full-page beautiful picture of an owl. We went to visit Dad's grave site on the way home. I took a printed picture of the kids and put it at the gravesite. As we approached the grave, I scanned the trees for an owl. Didn't see any.

When we got closer to the grave, much to my amazement, there was an ornamental owl sitting right on top of my Dad's tombstone. I did not remember this from the first time I visited the grave. It must have been there, but I did not have any connection to owls the last time I was there, so it did not register in my memory. It did this time, though! My higher power is giving me a clear signal.

I repeat, there was an owl on my Dad's tombstone. This entire owl experience is too much for me to ignore. Too much for me to chalk-up to pleasant co-incidence. I haven't shared this with anyone. It's too much to explain to others. Lindsay has an idea, but not really. My owl sightings are my earthly connection to a higher power. This is way too out there for the majority of people to understand. Most would think I'm crazy. I know I'm not crazy, so what is the use in trying to explain to others? It's my new supernatural belief. Like religion, it's best not to talk about it.

Aug 20, 2012– Journal Entry

We went camping as a family this weekend. I had a great time. On the first night camping, we stayed at a KOA in Revelstoke. We went to the pool and as we were walking there, Lindsay handed me her beer to hold while she adjusted something. As soon as I had the beer in my hand, I looked at a pond in front of me and there was a large ceramic Owl in the pond. I had walked by the pond at least three times prior to this, not noticing the owl. I also saw a painted owl on the KOA building as I was playing with Tylen, having fun. I take these owl sightings as messages that I'm on the correct path.

Oct 1, 2012– Journal Entry – 1 year sober

One year sober today. Allan celebrated his 10-year anniversary last night, and his topic was gratitude. Lindsay bought a block decoration that is on our kitchen windowsill that says, "Give thanks." The blocks have a small picture of an Owl on them. I

Red Pill in the Universal Matrix

went to a rehearsal of Annie tonight, which ended early, so I raced over to the Monday night AA meeting. I'm thankful for my life.

As I sat on the porch tonight, listening to the kids pick carrots from the garden, the setting sun hitting my face… I'm thankful I can derive so much pleasure from everyday moments. I'm thankful I appreciate the beauty of the world. I'm thankful that music makes me feel uplifted. I'm thankful my business is busy, my wife is happy, my kids are happy, I'm happy. I'm thankful I have friends. I'm thankful I've discovered that friends are not that important to my happiness. I'm thankful I've discovered my favorite thing to do is spend time with the kids. I'm thankful that I quit smoking weed. I'm thankful to have my confidence and happiness higher than it's ever been. I'm thankful that I don't worry about others not liking me anymore. I'm thankful that Lindsay has no problem with anything I do. I can pretty much do anything I want. I'm laughing more now. I am truly finding things funny. It's been years since this has happened. The kids make me laugh. I feel, with confidence, I'm headed down the right path. I thank AA. I thank my higher power. I thank my wife and friends.

Summary: Owls in the family

My first year sober was filled with synchronistic presentations of owls coming into my reality. The timing of the owls bolstered my belief that I was on the right path. The owls would manifest immediately before drinking situations or coupled with my own thoughts about drinking. They helped me stay sober when I needed to have faith in a higher power.

Here is a list of owl experiences. Some are almost trivial but were meaningful to me. Some are downright spooky.

- My kids and I visited my Dad's grave for the first time. It was the middle of a hot summer day…. A large owl was sitting on a low branch of a tree.
- Driving home from my second AA meeting, a large owl swooped in front of my car. That night, my old friend posted a picture of my Dad and me on Facebook.
- Before our big party, Shannon and Sierra came into the office and taught Sydney how to draw an owl. 2 large poster owls appeared before me, an hour before our party started.
- In Hawaii, In K-mart went into a trance looking at a display of hard alcohol bottles. I then proceeded to walk to the next aisle – books. I immediately picked up a book and it opened to a page with a picture of an owl. Then, randomly, I went to another page, another owl. That was spooky.
- Taking kids for a walk, I have an overwhelming feeling of love and happiness surge through me, bringing me to tears, looking at Brooklyn hiking through the woods, the sun shining through the trees, glistening off Brooklyn's hair. An overwhelming surge of positive emotion, love, and pure happiness coursed through my entire body. Like a finger of God reached out and surged love into my body. A few seconds later, a noise from behind me, an owl emerging from a tree right above me. That was incredible. That was a life-changing moment.
- I make the decision to quit smoking weed, and the day after, I go golfing with my high school buddies. They smoke weed through

the entire round. I say no thanks each time. On the 7th hole, four owls appear in the tree right beside the tee-off box.

- At Funtastic a few days later, driving everyone home at 1 am, Ashley asks me how I can be so patient. I contemplate how much fun I'm having, how calm I am, absolute serenity and pride and knowledge I'm doing the right thing…. an owl appears on a fence post next to the road.

- I take the kids camping in Osoyoos. Second visit to my Dad's grave. My Dad's grave has a decorative Owl on it. Something we did not take notice of the first time we visited.

The appearance of owls in my life opened my mind to the possibility of something other than nuts and bolts, a materialistic reality. I did not share the 'owlings' and how they guided me with anyone. It was too weird. It was not in line with my scientific-based reality. But it was my truth. It worked for me. Owls represented a massive synchronicity for me, before I knew what synchronicity was. When I got onto the path of not drinking, the synchronicities began. I did not consciously think about how the owls were steering me. Still, the owls came into my life exactly when I needed them and were responsible for partially opening my mind to something supernatural.

COVID 2020 and TikTok

My life between 2012 and 2020 was relatively normal. We worked and raised our kids, and nothing 'supernatural' occurred, as far as I could tell. I stayed sober from booze but ended up smoking weed again about a year after I quit. Nobody's perfect.

In 2020, COVID and the restrictions imposed hit me pretty hard. My business went from thriving and growing to nothing pretty much overnight. My focus for the past 20 years was no more. I had to lay off my employee. I struggled to find valuable tasks to do. My income vanished. I developed an addiction to TikTok. I was an early adopter of TikTok. I first tried TikTok to keep track of my kid's videos. But then I became curious as to how to make a video go 'viral' and I posted my first video. During the early days of the shutdown, I became obsessed with creating funny videos, gaining followers and creating videos the algorithm promoted. I was all about getting more views. More followers. I did some weird stuff.

At that time, the average age of the users of TikTok was teenagers. Few 'adults' were on the app. The exciting part of my storyline about TikTok is that it gave me the sense that I did not really care too much about what others thought of me. That being said if my clients were on the app, I'm not sure I would have done so many weird videos. I ended up having interactions with Charlie D'amelio and her Dad. Charlie D'amelio became the most viewed person on TikTok. Her Dad and I corresponded quite a bit, and we became Facebook friends.

At one point, when I had about 70,000 followers, I called a family meeting, and I sat everyone down at our dinner table and asked my family if they would be OK with being TikTok celebrities. I believed that being TikTok famous was possible and potentially lucrative, and I wanted to make sure I wasn't taking the family into a world we did not want to be in. Looking back on this, I find it humorous that I was so consumed by the app. It was part of my path, though. I gave careful consideration to being famous. I was not sure fame would be beneficial to the overall happiness of my family.

One time, when attending one of my daughter's basketball tournaments in Kamloops, a town about 2 hours from our hometown, there was a group of teenagers staring at me and taking pictures of me as I walked by in the hallway towards the gym. I knew they had seen my videos. Friends of my kids would come over, and they wanted to hang out with me because they were fans. One boy said my TikTok's helped him get through COVID. That felt good.

Eventually, as COVID dragged on, my ideas for creating funny TikTok videos started to dry up. The novelty and obsession started to waver, and my TikTok addiction fizzled.

Red Pill in the Universal Matrix

420 – April 20, 2021

On April 20, 2021, my friend Red and I met at the local golf course and smoked a joint to celebrate what has become an unofficial pot smokers' holiday in Canada, 420-day. Red and I had a few drinks, and then I had to pick up my daughter, Sydney, from the beach. Unbeknownst to me, it turned out that Sydney and her friends were also celebrating 420-day at the beach that evening. On the drive home, we were both a little more talkative than usual, but also both trying to hide our enthusiasm.

That night, I sat down at the TV and turned on the news show, 60 Minutes. I still watched the news back then. What I saw in that 60 Minutes episode changed my life forever. The story was on UAP's - Unidentified Aerial Phenomenon. "UFO" had been rebranded to "UAP" because there is a negative stigma associated with "UFO." That was the first time I had heard that term. I called Sydney down to the living room, and we re-watched the show together. It was a surreal night.

The reason I bring up 420 is because in 2022, when my reality started to really open up to something amazing, 420 was the first angel number that started appearing to me. Just like the owls came to me at key moments, the number 420 started coming into my life with strange coincidences attached. I'd wake up every morning at precisely 4:20 am without an alarm. I'd see 420 on websites, in work calculations, and I would always seem to check the time, exactly at 4:20 am and 4:20 pm. I also learnt that Elon Musk shares the same angel number. Something about the number 42 and this reality. It was weird. Here is my journal entry after seeing the 60 Minutes episode.

April 20, 2021 – Journal Entry

On 60 Minutes this week, they interviewed a US pilot who had a very compelling encounter with a tic-tac shaped UFO. I believed this guy, and I believed his co-pilot. I have now gone back and studied the unclassified UFO videos that have been verified by the US government. It is now crystal clear that there are several UFOs frequenting Earth every day. They have been for a very long time. They use a propulsion system that humans are not even close to being able to develop. When humans develop true AI, perhaps the AI will be able to create this technology. We also have UFO material in our procession, being studied. The US gov't is presenting a report in June. I feel like this information is simply not believed by the majority of people. I did not believe it until I saw the 60 Minutes episode. Regardless, I now believe, with verified evidence, that we are being visited from other planets. That means some type of speed of light travel is possible. That means there must be aliens from several other planets that are visiting us. It's possible we will be shown how to use the technology as soon as the aliens think we are safe enough to process it. If the aliens believe we are not mature enough or not safe enough to have this tech at our disposal, they won't let us get it. It's like the Americans will not let Iran get nuclear weapons. Or how humans don't give guns to monkeys. I feel like the first contact moment has happened to me. I'm in awe. We are not alone, and we have evidence of that. It's just a matter of time before others will realize. The full report is being released to the

US congress in June. I wonder how people will react if the information released is more compelling.

Apparently, the US government has considerably more compelling videos available, but they are trying to avoid panic by releasing too much. I feel like this should be the top news story. I feel like everything else is a distant second. We have alien technology buzzing in and out of our planet. What the fuck?! Why is this not the biggest news story of my lifetime? I'll tell you why people are afraid to admit they believe in aliens. Just like they are afraid to admit they are atheists – too much stigma. The videos and pilots' personal descriptions shown on 60 Minutes are ironclad proof. Alien tech is here. Done. Wow.

June 1, 2021 – Journal Entry

I've spent the last months trying to get the conversation going about the UFO issue with friends. I posted on Facebook and got zero responses. People don't really care. Or perhaps the issue is so far from their realm of reality that it's a non-starter. They simply think it's a hoax and don't consider it seriously.

I find these pilots to be professional, believable, and highly intelligent. The pilots exude integrity and I believe them 100%. They are telling us they encountered a flying object that flies 30 times faster than any human technology ever invented. Humans would be literally crushed by the g-forces created by this object. This has been confirmed by military radar, infrared scanners, the US government, Obama, and hundreds of US military. This means technology from a higher intelligence is frequenting Earth. Technology/Intelligence that far exceeds humans. This confirms that we are not alone in the universe. Why are we not talking about this?

My passion for the UFO topic started to ignite within me in the summer of 2021. But right as this new obsession started to blossom, the doldrums of COVID took hold of me.

COVID restrictions lasted so long. There was nothing to look forward to. Although I was excited about the possibility of extraterrestrial life after seeing the 60 Minutes episode, I was not aware of the amount of material available to study the topic. I was unaware of the books and podcasts or the community of people worldwide already interacting with higher intelligence. My passion for the unknown was lit on April 20th, but I had nothing to feed that passion. My friends were not interested. People just shunned the discussion, exactly like I would have done before seeing 60 Minutes.

With COVID robbing me of my business, my kid's sports, holidays and social interactions, I eventually became depressed. Then, a series of blows to our family put me into a tailspin. My thoughts were clouded with negativity. Anxiety. I saw my doctor for medication and a therapist to try and figure out how to get out of it. My journal entries from this period are scary to me, and I don't want to read them.

When I faced periods of depression and anxiety in my early life, I was able to remove myself from the situation and regroup. I would figure out what had gone wrong and go forward. That was not possible this time. My family meant everything to me, so I could not remove myself from the situation. I had to fight my way through it. I ended up essentially quitting my job, leaving my business for my employees to run. I took a job working as a painter. After two years of having little to do work-wise, this was a perfect move on my part. I needed that painting job. I needed some consistency. I needed a routine, and I needed to feel useful.

After working as a painter for a couple of months, my depression lifted, and in January 2022 I went back to working at my business. I was very fortunate to have an employee that kept my business running while I was falling to pieces. 2 years of COVID bullshit resulted in me having one of the biggest mental challenges I have ever faced. But with every valley, there is a peak. Life is all about peaks and valleys. I've come to believe that the challenges that we face serve a purpose. Life is all about learning lessons. 2022 turned out to be pretty much the most incredible year of my life. A complete change in my belief system. A tremendous spiritual awakening. A complete change in my understanding of the nature of this reality.

2022 – The Year of My Spiritual Awakening

As the COVID restrictions started to lift, life started getting back on track. My business started to get busy again, and I had stuff to do at work. My kids were able to play sports again. This meant the world to me. There was a light at the end of a very dark government restriction tunnel.

In early 2022, I started to feel elevated. Almost like I was in a minor manic stage, happy all the time. Eager to get up and read. I found the information related to UFOs so interesting, and I had decades of books and research to catch up on.

Jan 7, 2022 - Journal Entry

> I've been back working at Discovery for about the last month. The Christmas holidays were fun. Back at work… all good. Work is going well. My personal life is going well.
>
> I've been in communication with Allan [AA sponsor] lately. I have come to believe the universal matrix puts the right people in your path at the correct times. When Allan and I first met each other ten years ago, our first face-to-face meet-up was at a local restaurant. We were amazed to learn we were both adopted. We both grew up with white parents, and we both grew up unaware that our birth parents were of Native descent. Recently, Allan wrote a book, an autobiography. It's well-written and has a few pages dedicated to me, which was cool. The day he emailed the book to me for a pre-reading, I had an owl experience. The movie I was watching had an Owl in it, and the main character indicated

there is a connection between UFOs and Owls and said there is a book written about it. I am currently reading the book: "The Messengers: Owls, Synchronicity and the UFO Abductee." It turns out that owls and UFO sightings are closely linked. It turns out that thousands of others have had owls appear at amazing relevant times as well. Thousands of people have had UFO experiences, coupled with strange interactions with owls!

A book that combined my strange history of owls and my new UFO interest... was a good find. This book started me reading books on the topic of UFOs. It fed my new passion.

I also discovered many podcasts that deal with the UFO topic. Investigative journalists, and university professors, and Ph.D.s have been studying the 'Phenomenon' their whole lives. As I went down this rabbit hole, I consumed as much information as I could. Obsessed? Abso-fucking-lutely. When I get interested in something... I don't do it half-assed.

March 1, 2022 – Journal Entry

I've been feeling well for several months. I've completely stopped watching the news. I stopped listening to the New York Times podcast. I even change the station on the radio in the car if the news comes on. It's repulsive to me now. When I accidentally click on Google News and read a headline, I can feel my body physically react. I avoid the news completely. It is completely negative, ALL THE TIME. I don't need that. Nobody needs that.

As I began reading and listening to audiobooks, my knowledge increased. My mind started putting things together, connecting some dots, and I learnt the US Air Force has been hiding reality from citizens since WWII. My mind opened. I was awakened to several different possibilities of what we are dealing with when it comes to UFOs. For me, my awakening began with an interest in the topic of UFOs. I learnt a new term for coincidence: **synchronicity**. I also realized that my life was starting to be loaded with synchronicities.

March 12, 2022 – Journal Entry

It's 5 am on a Saturday morning. I am waking up earlier with a lot of energy lately. I realized something this morning. It's possible that I have stumbled upon the nature of our reality. Have you ever really stopped to think of the absolute heaven that Earth is? In almost every sci-fi movie that has another planet with sentient beings, none of those planets are better than Earth. If I were to create my own planet for humans to live on, I don't think I could imagine a better planet than Earth.

The human race is very close to giving birth to a new life form – Artificial General Intelligence (**AGI**). This might come by merging human biology with AGI. OR it might come with AGI developing all on its own.

AGI will be millions of times more intelligent than all humans combined in a short period of time. 90% of AI experts feel strongly that this transition will happen before 2040. AGI could happen much sooner. Elon Musk believes it will happen by 2026. Humans will be intellectual slugs compared to AGI. Way down on the food chain.

The next part of the journal entry was a result of some of the books I had read up to that date. It is not what I believe now, but it was part of my process of awakening to the nature of this reality.

Other species in the Universe have already developed AGI. These species have a firm grasp on the nature of reality in our universe.

These entities have mastered interstellar travel, and they can control the consciousness of lower life forms (animals and humans to some extent). Higher Intelligent Beings (HIB) have been interacting with humans for at least 70000 years. Around 70000 years ago, HIB tweaked human biology, accelerating our capacity for intelligence. Earth was a perfect garden and the HIB fertilized humans. Why would they do that? Why not just land on Earth and start living here? It's a beautiful planet. Maybe they did. Maybe an asteroid or an ice age sent the HIB's packing. Maybe they still live on Earth. Maybe they live inside Earth, under the oceans.

Technology is advancing faster than we can keep track of. We are evolving infinitely fast. It will surpass humans in intelligence soon. We will have to merge with computers to be relevant. I'm sure that other planetary species have gone down the same path. That path leads to a strange hybrid computer/living future.

Aliens abduct humans. Not sure how often but they do. During abduction, the aliens are perceived to get samples, sperm, babies, etc. Maybe in the future, sex becomes obsolete. The networked computer mind is the future life form. They still need some living beings to get things done. Grays are just hive mind droids that serve the higher intelligence. The higher intelligence needs Grays to interact with the 3D world.

Manifestation – The Secret

Before 2022, I had never heard of manifestation. Manifestation is the process of visualizing a future event and then the imagined event manifests in real life. For example, I visualized my son smiling after a hockey game. In my head, I pictured him smiling, and I felt the happy emotions that seeing Tylen happy brings to me. It turned out, at hockey practice that week, after my smile visualization, Tylen's coaches taught Tylen how to use his body and get positioning on the other team's defense.

Tylen ended up playing one of the best games of his life and he won the MVP for the game. My wife Lindsay took a picture of Tylen with the MVP medallion around his neck and a huge smile. I had actually forgotten my visualization of the smile on Tylen's face until Lindsay sent me the picture. It was awesome. Visualize a positive future event, and the event will manifest in your reality.

Before my spiritual awakening, the description of manifestation and how our excited thoughts somehow manifest in this 3D physical reality… that would be a non-starter for me. It sounds like utter nonsense. How could visualizing a future reality in your head, somehow materialize in real life?? When you are an atheist, believing in evolution and a nuts-and-bolts reality, manifestation is not a possibility. But as I started to follow the path the universe was putting in front of me, it was clear manifestation worked, somehow. Even if you have not heard about it or believe in it, manifestation works. Interestingly, when people pray, they will tell the universe what they want. Sometimes these prayers are coupled with visualizations of future events. In order for this to be possible, somehow, our thoughts have to be connected to the universe. Our thoughts have to somehow be connected to the intelligence generating this reality.

It was very interesting how the Universe arranged for me to learn about 'The Secret.' It happened in March 2022 when we were attending Basketball provincials. My daughter Brooklyn had played with the same team of friends since grade 6. The team qualified for BC Provincials in Grade 8, Grade 10 and Grade 12. In Grade 11, COVID cancelled all basketball games. This group of girls fought through the adversity of COVID restrictions and kept practicing. In Grade 12, my other daughter, Sydney, joined the team.

After two years of COVID hell, a few weeks before the provincial finals, the province of BC allowed spectators to attend sporting events again. What an incredible experience to be allowed back into the gym to watch again. It brings tears to my eyes to think of the joy of watching my daughters play on the same team. But this was Brooklyn's final year. As parents, we had supported the team through many ups and downs and twists and it came down to this final provincials tournament.

On the final night before our last game, we gave the girls a sendoff banquet in the team hotel restaurant. It was a great night. This group of parents knew this would be the last time we had a chance to party together. 6 of us ended up back in our hotel room. Everybody was feeling no pain. I was chatting with one of the Dads, and he started to tell me about how his football coach in college had the entire team lie on their backs and visualize executing plays and positive outcomes. This Dad was a particularly close talker.

Perhaps the closest talker I have ever encountered in my entire life. He kept on getting up from the couch and coming over to the chair I was sitting in and talking to me, centimeters' away from my face. It was odd. I had to push him back a few times and told him to sit back on the couch. He was just extremely enthusiastic about whatever he was talking about. I chalked it up to booze. But it was the third time he came back to talk to me, face-to-face, that he told me about the book, 'The Secret'. When somebody is talking that close to you, you have no choice but to pay attention.

At the time, I did not think too much about the book recommendation, but within a few weeks, I had purchased the audiobook and started listening to it while walking in the woods. It was life-changing. So many reputable life coaches, psychologists and celebrities all preaching about the same amazing characteristic of this reality. The book changed my life.

Since then, I have read many books on manifestation. Taken online courses. I've run tests that have manifested. Essentially, you have to imagine a future scene in your head. You really have to imagine it to the point where you can feel the emotions associated with that outcome. If your manifestation is within the realm of the possible, and it truly excites you or makes you feel intense love or some other positive emotion, this miraculous reality will make that wish come true. I know it sounds crazy. But it is fucking real.

When I think back to my own life, without knowing it, I have always been someone who chases after my passions. I'm an all-or-nothing type. In grade 11, my first year attending Vernon Secondary School, I heard there was a ping pong team that practiced at lunch. I went out to give it a try. I really liked it. I had never really played ping pong or owned a ping pong table, but this seemed like a fun lunchtime activity. I built a ping pong table that we could put on top of our pool table at home. I practiced by myself for hours every night. I improved quickly, and in Grade 12 I qualified to be 1 of the 3 players on the team.

Our school hosted the provincial championship in grade 12 and my team got third place in the province. I didn't care what people thought of me. Table tennis was not exactly a chick magnet sport. I even had a girl from another school stop talking to me when a picture of our ping pong team ended up in the sports section of our local paper. Table tennis was fun, and I was good at it. Follow your passion. If something excites you and elevates your happiness, even a little bit, follow that excitement. That is an absolute rule of this reality. That is how you find your true path.

Even though I did not know about manifestation, my passions made my goals manifest. The one big one was my current house. When I read the Tony Robbins book in 2013, I was able to identify my goal of living in a house with an amazing view. I have really been dreaming about views my entire life. I estimated it would take ten years to accomplish this goal. Three years later, we purchased a 23-acre lot with one of the best views in Canada.

The realtor had named the lot "Fantasia." Fantasia was listed for sale for 8 years and nobody bought it. I used to walk with my kids on the land before it was developed. I have loved views my entire life. Views excite me. It is the way I was wired when I dropped down into existence. Was I lucky that everything worked out the way it did? I don't think it was luck at all. I think my passion for views manifested the opportunity and I followed my

Red Pill in the Universal Matrix

passion. I was fortunate the Tony Robbins book was put in my path. Tony Robbins is completely aware of manifestation. So is Oprah and Jim Carrey. So are a lot of very successful people. It's a cheat code to success in this reality.

One of the rules about manifesting is that if your manifestations are for the greater good, they are more likely to manifest. I don't think you can manifest things that hurt others or decrease the overall happiness of others. Much better to manifest stuff that helps others.

How can our excited thoughts actually become things in the world? How the fuck does that actually happen?

March 14, 2022 – Journal Entry

> I'm listening to the audiobook, "The Secret." There have been times in my life where my happy thoughts have manifested reality. Was this the universe pulling strings? Was my deceased father making these things happen? Are the rules of this reality governed by consciousness?

> To summarize, humans create our Earth's reality through our thoughts. If we live in a matrix-like simulation, there must be some rules that govern the direction the simulation goes. Positive emotionally charged thoughts can steer the direction of the simulation. What emotions is the simulation trying to maximize? Gratitude. Things that generate gratitude are more likely to manifest.

Redtastic:

One of the suggestions for readers of 'The Secret' was to test out manifesting something into reality. So I decided to follow the directions of the book and attempt to manifest a **red** balloon. That night, me and my son, Tylen were driving to pick up Brooklyn from work. I told Tylen we would do a test to manifest a red balloon. As we were driving through town that evening, looking for red balloons, something strange happened to me. Things that were red were really standing out. I mean really standing out. Like nothing before in my life, the colour red was almost like it was illuminated to me. It was interesting. Two days later, in a TikTok video about the future of fast food that 'randomly' came into my video stream, there were red balloons. Not a huge manifestation but it opened my mind a tiny bit. Something about the colour red is telling me to appreciate my life. It's hard to describe. The colour red makes me feel connected and appreciative. I've never had a favourite colour before. Now red is catching my attention everywhere.

Yesterday on the walk, I was listening to The Secret audiobook. I listened to the chapter dedicated to manifesting wealth. Determine what money you want, and feel the excitement that money will bring to your life. Really feel it. On the walk, I determined I wanted $5 million. About 10 minutes later, a bird almost landed on me. The bird came branch by branch closer to me, stared at me, and did not fly away. I even moved. I could have reached out and touched the bird for at least 10 seconds. As he moved, branch by branch closer to me… I honestly thought it was going to land on me. I continued the walk, happy, feeling connected to the Universe. I ended up putting music on and dancing. Singing. Joyful. I saw something red on the walk and I felt joyous. 30 seconds later, I looked down and saw a $5 bill, sitting perfectly in the middle of the path. I've spent probably 100's of hours walking, on 100's of days and I have never found money.

The $5 note made me awe inspired. When I got home, I wrote a cheque for myself, just like Jim Carrey did when he was younger. I reached in my office cupboard to get the cheque and onto my desk fell a red keepsake item that my birth mother, Yvonne gave me. The keepsake actually looks like a red balloon. I phoned Yvonne for the first time in a few years. Life is interesting….

April 9, 2022 – Journal Entry

Had an incredible experience with Allan, my AA sponsor. I've been sober for ten years. Allan and I have lost contact, but we will email a couple of times per year. On April 9, I emailed him a picture of a rainbow. The rainbow was a symbol of Allan's spiritual awakening 20 years prior. Here is the exchange below. I did not know the significance of the timing of my email. Just a coincidence. I emailed a picture of a rainbow to Allan and here is his response:

From: Allan

Sent: April 8, 2022 2:49 PM

Subject: Re: Rainbow

This is so awesome! And perfect timing. When I first had my major rainbow experience I had asked God for a rainbow to come sometime before my birthday. It came the day before my birthday, on the drive home from a birthday dinner with my mom. It just so happens that today is the day before my birthday.

Thank you for sending this. Made my day!

Allan

April 15, 2022 – Journal Entry

On Saturday, April 9, we went to my friend Red's house for a dinner party, and they were dog-sitting. A nice little dog. I had a revelation that I secretly told each of the partygoers that evening: the Lewis's are going to get a dog. I told everyone in attendance except Lindsay. I felt strongly that my son Tylen needed a dog. *Problem:* Lindsay has always been strongly against having a dog. I did not tell Lindsay about my secret plan to get a dog. I needed to have my family and Lindsay's sisters on my side before talking to Lindsay about a dog. On Monday, I spoke to Tylen and Brooklyn and got them both excited about it. Syd does not like dogs. Brooklyn started texting me pics and videos of dogs. On Wednesday, I spoke to Lindsay's sisters and their husbands, eliciting their help and future dog-sitting services. I did all this planning behind Lindsay's back. I was planning on telling Lindsay at the right time. My words to Lindsay's sister, I will tell Lindsay after she has had 3 beers – the perfect timing was key. On Friday, April 15, 6:30 pm, Lindsay went for a walk above our house by herself. She came around the corner, and in the middle of the trail was a French bulldog, asleep. Shocked, Lindsay attempted to pet the little guy, but the dog was scared. It ran from her toward our house. She followed, and she enlisted the help of Tylen. They attempted to find the little dog, but he disappeared.

I had spent the week planning behind Lindsay's back, getting my troops in line for the solid front I planned to present to Lindsay. The dog manifested on the path for Lindsay. Just like the $5 note, we have never had a dog appear on the paths above our house. When Lindsay came and told me about the dog on her path, I told her everything about how I had planned to get a dog all week. Later that night, a post on Lindsay's Facebook feed showed the missing dog. The dog's name was Brutus. It had run away from the dog park in the middle of Vernon that afternoon. It ran all the way across Vernon, up the mountain, into the woods and then proceeded east towards Lumby. This is a small-legged dog. It appears he ran out of energy on our path, right above our house. He lay down to rest right on the path Lindsay walked on. Am I suggesting something steered Brutus to this exact point on the path? Yes, I believe that. From that point forward, I believed I could manifest things.

A funny side story: Lindsay represents Julius Caesar. I'm the Roman Senators plotting behind her back, organizing the assassination of her anti-dog stance. Brutus was the final knife in the back of my plan to overtake Caesar. Et tu Brute? Et tu? Another instant in my life where I have hidden the truth and I have been found out quickly.

April 18, 2022 – Journal Entry

On Saturday, April 16, we had a few friends over and we went for a walk. On this walk, one of my friends disclosed that she had a paranormal event occur to her while on vacation in Mexico. She woke up in the middle of the night, from a deep sleep, with a dark entity choking her. It was a dark shadowy figure that left when she fought it off. Of course, she was terrified and woke up her husband in panic. She is 100% certain that this was no dream. Horrifying.

I started a new book on Monday evening (Apr 20). This is a book I had downloaded a month prior to me hearing about my friend's horrible story. It turns out that her experience is common. In the book, a Harvard Professor, John E. Mac, becomes interested in studying the Phenomenon when the exact same experience that my friend had, happened to him. I could not believe that the book I was listening to, written by a New York Times Reporter, had a very clear description of exactly what my friend had told me two days earlier. I shared the information with her and she found it helpful to know that she was not alone. Here is an excerpt taken from the book:

"David Hufford, a PhD and a professor at Pennsylvania State College of Medicine, joined the conference and came to share what he knew, which was the phenomenon of awakening paralyzed in the presence of a malevolent being. He had, to his terror, unaccountably experienced it himself as a student in the 1960s, after which he had gone on to study the experience in Newfoundland, where it was surprisingly prevalent and known as

Red Pill in the Universal Matrix

the old hag syndrome, nocturnal visitations by an evil presence, is seemingly bent on strangling or suffocating immobilized victims."

The coincidence of this coming up in my book 2 nights after my friend's disclosure… something is guiding these synchronicities.

April 19, 2022 – Journal Entry

In the past few weeks, the synchronicities in my life have been coming fast and furious. I'm reading "Dying to be Me" by Anita Moorjani. This is a lady who had a miraculous Near Death Experience (NDE), and she came back with incredible knowledge about the nature of reality.

Yesterday, on page 159, I read this passage in the book:

Living in harmony with who we truly are means being and doing things that make us happy, things that arouse our passion and bring out the best of us, things that make us feel good – and it also means loving ourselves unconditionally. When we're flowing in this way and feeling upbeat and energized about life, we're in touch with our own magnificence. When we can find that within us, things really start getting exciting, and we find synchronicities happening all around us.

Well, the synchronicities are definitely happening around me. This morning, Tyler Henry, a very powerful psychic medium, followed me on Twitter. Tonight, I reached out to Peggy and told her about this because I was proud to have this prominent medium follow me. Peggy has been a life-long friend of ours. She is a psychic medium. I've never believed in the powers of psychics. I've never thought anyone could be connected to another world. I'm now changing that belief. Something is interacting with my reality. Things are changing.

Thursday, April 20, 2022 – Journal Entry

Recently I've become considerably more open to the possibility that some sort of afterlife. I just finished an incredible book about near-death experiences. In the next life, all time is right now. No time. Everything is happening right now. You pretty much have infinite knowledge as it relates to anything to do with Earth based you.

Well, this is getting pretty awesome…. another day, another amazing synchronicity. Barry, my Godfather, took over as my father figure and the Grampa to our kids after my Dad passed away. Barry was an amazing man and lifelong family friend. He passed away about 5 years ago. When Barry passed away, I was the executor of his will. Now that I am very open to the possibility of my loved ones still existing in another realm, I felt like when I was given the responsibility of managing Barry's affairs when he passed; I handled my interaction with Barry's long-term landlord selfishly. Not like Barry would have wanted me to. I bartered with the landlord about the rent payable for Barry's vacant condo, after Barry passed. My actions felt morally wrong. I know Barry would not approve. I felt guilty. The next day, we could no longer get Netflix to work on Barry's iPad, which we were still using as our video screen to watch Netflix on our treadmill. I tried to fix it and get it working, but I do not know the password for Barry's Apple ID. I did know it at one point. It was written down. I took the iPad to the office and opened up Barry's file with all the paperwork I had on Barry. There, in the file, was the email address of the landlord. I felt compelled to email the landlord and apologize. So I did. I hope he got the email. He did not reply. I hope it provided some closure to him. I still could not find the iPad Apple password, and I still could not get Netflix to work on the iPad. That evening, I tried again, and for some reason, Netflix continued to work. This could be a stretch, but it is a coincidence involving my thoughts of guilt about Barry, and an electronic malfunction steering me to the action needed. After the apology, the iPad works again.

April 26, 2022 – Journal Entry

Yesterday we interviewed an awesome applicant for our next project manager at my work. She will be hired and she will be instrumental in helping our business grow.

As I was getting ready to go into the office to interview her, I was a bit stressed dealing with the kids in the house right before the interview. As I was trying to go out the front door of our house and walk over to my detached home office, Sydney stopped me and insisted on giving me something. She gave me a ceramic owl she made at school. It had taken her months to make. The teacher kept forgetting to put the owl in the kiln. Literally seconds before meeting an important part of the future of my business, the universe presented me with an owl. When I walked outside to the office, I could hear the applicant's vehicle as she arrived for her interview. Of course, we hired her. I feel so much gratitude to the universe. I love this life. THANK YOU.

April 27, 2022 – Journal Entry

I've been getting up early these days, around 5 am, because I'm so excited and eager to get going on a new day. I have so much information I want to take in. Last evening, another incredible occurrence. Dropped off Tylen at baseball practice. I proceeded to listen to the UFO podcast with Luis Elizondo. INSPIRING. Love it. Went to the car wash. Cleaned out the inside of my car. Went to the gas station at the Superstore.

The lady filling up beside me started conversing with me about how much gas was. Very friendly exchange that ended with me saying we are in crazy times right now. She agreed. I then went to the Superstore feeling charged. I noticed a number of people that gave me smiles. One lady was quite far from me, passing at the end of the aisle. She saw me and smiled at me big time, and it actually caught me off guard. I smiled back and tried to figure out if I had known her. It seemed like the happiness I felt was contagious to people around me.

As I was checking out, I was asked by the cashier if I wanted the deal of the day, I said no thanks. The older lady bagging her groceries in front of me said, "You mean you don't want a wooden spoon?" She then proceeded to instigate a conversation about how she used to use wooden spoons to discipline her kids. I contributed with, my mom broke a wooden spoon on me growing up. The lady stated, "You can't hit kids these days."

Throughout my life I have told only one story about my mom, how she broke a wooden spoon on my butt when I was five years old. The wooden spoon was the one topic that would excite the neurons in my brain to think of my mom.

I then drove to Don Cherry's, a local pub. I was meeting with some of my 'Tuesday night' friends, but I was early. I parked, put in my Airpods, listening to a podcast and proceeded to walk around the parking lot. I ended up sitting on the far side of the empty parking lot, completely consumed by the podcast. Completely inspirational podcast about the Phenomenon.

I noticed that an elderly woman was making her way toward me. She made a decision to visit me because it was a long walk across the empty parking lot. She arrived and sat down beside me on the cement stairs I was sitting on. We proceeded to chat. Her name was Maureen, my mom's sister's name. In the conversation that followed, I spoke about happy times from my past, on a train with my father. I spoke of happy times with Lindsay on the graduation field trip to Calgary. I spoke of UFOs, Elon Musk, and driverless cars, and I bonded with this lovely old lady. Maureen spoke of her life growing up with a father who worked for the railroad. Railroad people are like family, she said. My grandfather worked for the railroad, and this created a very interesting conversation.

Eventually, I noticed Maureen was wearing a bracelet, and we looked at it and determined it was a bracelet from the Vernon Hospital. I asked her if she sleeps at the hospital sometimes. She said yes. She was a long way from the hospital.

I asked her if it would be a good idea to perhaps go check with the hospital to see if she was supposed to be there. She said yes. She was happy that I owned a Toyota because she owned a Toyota and was happy to get into a very clean car. I drove her to the hospital and the nurses were very thankful that I brought her back. She had wandered away from the hospital in the afternoon and ended up in my path on the other side of town. She walked up to the right person.

When I woke up this morning, Lindsay said she felt this exchange with Maureen was my mom coming to me. I must admit, I've been thinking about my mom more than ever lately. The wooden spoon connection was really a fortunate coincidence. The song, 'Jolene' by Dolly Parton was a song that my mom liked. I've replaced 'Jolene' with Maureen and I have been singing it this morning.

April 28, 2022 – Journal Entry

Woke up at 4:20 am this morning. I did not set an alarm; I just woke up at 4:20 am. Started to think about a new goal… **climbing the tallest mountain in BC.** Lindsay and I will retire and train for mountain climbing adventures. That seems exciting. Anyway, lying in bed…I continued to think… I determined a new task; what I thought I was meant to do. I was charged up, lying in bed,

Red Pill in the Universal Matrix

thinking about this new goal: I want to give speeches at high schools introducing the most important scientific discovery in the history of mankind… the Phenomenon. Excited, I got up for the day and walked toward our on-suite bathroom.

At the exact moment I passed under the fire alarm in our bedroom, it beeped. Has it beeped ever before? No. Did any of the other fire alarms in our house beep? No. It appears the backup battery for our bedroom fire alarm gave up at that exact moment… immediately after, the very exciting thought came into my head and exactly when I was underneath the fire alarm. I stopped in my tracks, looked directly up and knew instantly what had occurred. The universe is guiding me, giving me signposts in the form of synchronicities. I'm thankful for this universe, intelligence, God, Barry, Mom, Dad, Russ and everyone else who is invested in my well-being. Thank you.

===Same day…. That night…..

Turned on Amazon Prime. Started to scroll and stopped on "The Mystery Mountain Project Documentary" and started watching. Looked good. Paused it. Went upstairs to get snacks. Came back and pressed play to find out the movie was about the first people that hiked the tallest mountain in BC. Yeah, that is correct; the same day, I woke up and typed my journal entry saying I wanted to hike the tallest mountain in BC… I randomly chose to watch a movie about the first people to climb the tallest mountain in BC. Thank you.

Red Pill in the Universal Matrix

Friday, April 29, 2022 – Journal Entry

Made my appointment with Peggy, our friend with a connection to something beyond this reality. I shared with Peggy the people's names who I think are important to me on the other side: Mom, Dad, Barry and Russ. We set the appointment for May 4 at 9:30 am. May the 4th be with you.

The same morning, 30 minutes later, at about 10 am, Lindsay and I watched two quails fight all across our backyard. I went outside to watch. Then the strangest thing happened. The winning quail walked directly to the edge of our balcony and followed me around the corner onto the front balcony. It was odd. It was really cool to have this beautiful little bird on our balcony. It would walk right up to you.

Saturday April 30, 2022 – Journal Entry

John came over for a 7:30 am walk. John is a new friend. Someone that came into my path at the exact right time. John was my daughter's basketball coach this season. Both my daughters played on the Sr. Girls Basketball team. So did John's daughter.

Right when I was learning so much about the "Phenomenon," I was eager to share with those around me, and I told some very hard-to-believe stories to some of the other basketball parents and coaches on a tournament trip to Vancouver. Everybody was polite, but I could see the 'what is this guy on' looks that others were exchanging.

On our next basketball trip to Vancouver, I was reading a book in the mall while the girls shopped. John came and sat with me and presented an open-minded attitude about what I was talking about related to the Phenomenon. It turned out that John grew up in a household that was connected to some type of higher intelligence.

When John was a child, a spaceship landed in the field right by his farm, and his entire family came outside and saw the craft and the beings that came out of the strange disk-shaped UFO. His background and personal experiences matched so many of the accounts I had been reading about. On our walk that Saturday morning, John disclosed to me that the story he told me on our last walk, he had not talked about or thought about for decades. He has shut off memories of earlier points in his life. It was the story about a demonic holographic face coming out of the wall that he and his siblings and friends were very petrified by. John's Dad had to climb on the other side of the stair railing to smash the glass panel that had a holographic entity coming out of it. Very scary for him and his young siblings and friends.

I'm very connected to John. He is not judgmental. On our walks, we talk about the evidence that is available, him from his entire family's personal experiences and me from the small library of books and multiple podcasts I have ferociously consumed lately. He is completely in line with me on this path. Open-minded. We walked for at least 2 hours when we ended up on a path I have never been on and we came across a rare flower, a chocolate lily. I stopped to take a picture, and I told John these were Lindsay's favorite flowers. I told him that Lindsay almost channels her father, Russ, when she is looking at nature. The way she gets excited about wild asparagus and other rare flowers that we come across our path when walking… this is exactly like her Russ was. Right at this exact moment, a huge owl flew out of a tree right over the top of us and landed in another tree right beside our path. The owl stopped and looked at us and then flew right back to us and landed on another tree. It was an amazing owl and we saw it clear as day. Signpost… yes. Thank you so much. To be honest, I'm not completely sure who I'm saying thank you to anymore. At this point, I feel like MOM, DAD, RUSS, and BARRY are all working to help me. I love this life. I've created a Spotify playlist called "My Team" and filled it with songs that remind me of my deceased loved ones. When I listen to these songs, I feel emotionally elevated and connected to my spiritual team.

Last night, someone on Twitter sent me a YouTube video about the Monroe Institute and remote viewing and essentially the meaning of life. Being able to intentionally instigate an out-of-body experience. Everything about this video fits with everything I have been learning about. It will be interesting to try it out.

Sunday, May 1, 2020 – Journal Entry

Luis Elizondo and Sean Cahill appeared on the Zed podcast. They are going to explain how consciousness is related to the Phenomenon. All my instincts tell me that this is the beginning of true disclosure. I've been given the knowledge to recognize that this is important. Am I crazy? No, not at all. Am I emotionally charged because I feel like I'm close to being exposed to a new reality… 100%. So many sources have indicated to me that the human body is just the crust of existence. True life is within our consciousness.

We have had the quail on our balcony for three days straight. I feel like this is another synchronicity put before me. Peggy calls the bird a spirit messenger. I feel my mom's spirit is strong. I feel Russ's spirit is strong. I have a team of love behind me. Showing a path forward. I need to figure that path out, and my spiritual Team is trying to guide me. Thank you.

May 2, 2020 – Journal Entry

Last night, I went in the back yard and sat with Trish the quail – our new pet. My mom, Trish, died of lung cancer when I was 19 years old.

On my TikTok feed… Jeff Bezos was working in a very well-paid job when he quit to start Amazon. He said to himself he would not be happy on his deathbed if he looked back, not having taken that chance. I read a book that essentially says find your passion, find the things that excite you, and somehow make that passion into your profession. When I woke up at 4:20 am with the powerful thought that I needed to give speeches about the Phenomenon…. and the fire alarm beeped. That was a transcendent message sent to me. At this point, I need to continue to get my business to grow. I then need to figure out how to spread the word and spread my knowledge about the Phenomenon. There needs to be a business I can set up that helps people. It appears that remote viewing and the different types of consciousness are in the future. I'm not certain how to merge my passion with a profession yet, but it's pretty certain that if I can do it... I can live in an elevated state, merging my passion with helping people. I've been waking up so early lately. Charged to start the day. Mom, Dad, and anyone else connected to my well-being... if you can make this path happen for me... that would be appreciated. Show me how I can mix my passion with my profession. Put me on the path that maximizes my happiness and helps people. Thank you.

May the fourth – Journal Entry

Today, I have my session with Peggy. I've been completely awestruck at how the universe is putting things in my path. Trish is hugely present. Last evening, I texted John and established that he was ok with continuing to be a friend and support mechanism as we go through this journey. As the sun was setting, I walked up the mountain behind our house, and I put on my Mom's favourite song, "Stand by Your Man," and cried and danced and sang. Feeling my mom inhabit me, joyous. Higher vibration. Elevated. I then walked a bit and noticed a rainbow circling the sun. I danced all across the mountain. Joyous. Pure joy. Sat and enjoyed the sun in one of the many chairs I have set up on the mountain. Felt like I was with Mom, Dad, Barry, Russ and a powerful group of souls supporting me and my family.

The quail has been living at our house. It stares into our house. It follows me to the office when I'm not in the house. I have googled this... this is not a behavior that birds exhibit. This is my mom somehow controlling this little bird. Ha ha. That is a pretty incredible statement.

Today, I had an urge to stare at myself in the mirror. Not sure where this urge came from. I stared for about 2 minutes, but nothing happened. I then went out into the living room and turned on TikTok. The first video that came up was a guy recommending that you stare at yourself in the mirror, which is exactly what I had just done. I've noticed incredible synchronicities within TikTok and Reels feeds. The other side appears to have control of the social media feeds we see. Or it can control my thinking, and it knows what is coming in my path.

This morning, I will have my session with Peggy. I'm hoping she will receive as clear of a message as she can possibly receive. I know something is happening. I'm grateful for this. I'm living in an amazing universe.

Peggy Reading 1:

Peggy is a psychic medium. She has the ability to connect with intelligence outside of this reality. For as long as I've known Peggy, 30+ years, I did not believe anything like this could be possible. But given the events leading up to my first reading, I knew my reality was being influenced by something.

Peggy did not ask me any questions. She did not ask me to provide any questions. We did not even meet face to face. I did not give Peggy any indication of what I was hoping for from this reading. She did ask me to share the names and birthdays of the people in my life that have passed.

People who might want to connect with me. I gave her my Mom, Dad, Barry and Russ. We set a date and time, and Peggy instructed me to be in a quiet place, be relaxed, and be open to anything that comes to me. I was at home, and Peggy was on the other side of the city in her home. I decided to walk up the mountain and essentially meditate during the half-hour reading.

As I sat there, surrounded by nature, I thought back to joyous times I could remember. I was emotional. At the end of the half-hour, Peggy called me to tell me what had come through. The first message that she received was that "I am an anomaly." She received messages from all my spiritual team. It all rang true to me. Peggy gave me messages from my Mom that there was no possible way Peggy could have made up. She recited a perfect description of the relationship that my Mom and I had, the type of kid I was from my Mom's perspective. It was mind-blowing. She confirmed that my spiritual team was making adjustments to this reality to help our family. A lot of tears were shed. To me, this reading was just another domino in the string of supernatural miracles that seemed to be happening to me all the time. It bolstered my love for my spiritual team.

I've recommended Peggy's services to many people, but I have found that you have to be open and ready to accept this type of communication from loved ones who have passed. Here is the summary that Peggy emailed me after the reading:

Cale, there is so much more to this than you realize. You are an anomaly. You see, each moment, each person who has entered and exited your life has been with purpose, growth and intention. You are only now realizing the immense scope of it. That is the tip of the iceberg, really. How wide are your eyes willing to be opened? How much are you willing to see? Absorb? Understand? Your capacity and willingness are matched by your capability and understanding to know, see, and feel the truth. Are you really ready?

There is a reason you changed locations so many times growing up. There is also a reason you searched for your birth parents. You learned how to adapt. You know how to adapt. Your brain is literally magnetic and expanding.

Yes, the answer is yes, the Owl is me, Dad. He had been trying to get through to you for a long time. You had noticed subtle things, but you did not pay attention to them. Don't forget, my son, the end of life - is only just the beginning. And him using the phrase 'my son' was not something he used liberally - he really meant it. You were, and you always will be, his son (Awe!) He has fierce pride and love for you, emotions and tears in his eyes, which he fiercely wipes away. You have made him proud beyond belief, and he says, "You have outdone yourself, Cale.' He and the others are protectors of your children. Although believe it or not – sometimes Russ gets protective over 'his' girls.

Cale, you are the one they left behind. You are so much more than what meets the eye – and you know this, and you are coming into your own now. Literally, your true self. The way will become clear to you. Be open. Receptive and in love, light, and truth. ALWAYS.

I feel like your Dad is a quiet man who kept to himself and did not express himself. Hmmm, it's like he's in a corner – weird, like a boxing match or a ring. Ha – the word for Russ is territorial – not protective – well, that too, but territorial with Barry. Lol. They are chums. Sometimes, they argue about who's intervening or doing or saying what – it's a friendly banter between them.

Your mom, Trish, says, you never needed me, Cale. You were always so busy in your head. She was always there and still is, but she knew, deep down, that you never really needed her. You were always independent on your own path. She was like your silent cheerleader mom. (Awe). Trish is with you. She has her hand out on your right shoulder. She loves you in the most nurturing, motherly way. She sees now you really did need her, but you pretended you didn't try and ease the burden of her illness and passing. Awe... truth. She loves you and is with you now. It's Ok to still need her. You are healing the mother wound from all directions. And she is sorry, she knew it would be hard – her leaving. She feels your disappointment. Her hand is on your heart now, purple love and healing. Filling you.

Cale, you will go to the moon! Whether physically as you really want to or energetically. You WILL. You achieve everything you put your mind to. Always have. Now it's time to put your body, mind and soul into it combined – and you will create miracles. You already are. We are pleased and proud of you. Always.

All avenues lead to your whole experience; don't discount any – you are missing some, Barry says, like pieces of the puzzle; find them, call them, and integrate them into all of your experiences on Earth. ALL parts matter! You know you have been coded, right? (I don't know what that means) but it's for you to know and understand. And you already do. You jumped up with high vibrational energy.

What you have to understand is that Peggy never met my Mom and Dad. I'm friends with Peggy but before this reading, she really had no insight into what I have been experiencing in my real life. She had no idea about my relationship with my Mom; nobody did.

The message that came through to Peggy was exactly what I needed at the time. I came away from the reading with 100% certainty that the Mom and Dad were able to communicate through Peggy. That is an incredible feeling. The parental pride that I craved my entire life is still being felt by those on the other side of this temporary, earth-bound existence.

May 6 – 2022 – Journal Entry

> The quail has been living on our front deck all week. Every morning, I go out on the deck before work and broadcast the quail on my Facebook live feed. I've cleaned up its poop. I really feel my mom is the spirit behind this quail. At lunch, I came in from the office and sat with the quail on the front deck. That afternoon, Lindsay thought I was getting a bit weird in my relationship with the quail. Rightfully so. Some people came over to our house that night. So, after a week of living with the quail on our front patio, I announced to the sky, "Mom, thank you for the quail, but it's time for the quail to move on and live a normal life." The next day, the quail was gone.

May 11, 2022 – Journal Entry

Yesterday, I walked up to a homeless person and gave him $40. He had a red hat on. Red is my colour. Funny, I have a strange feeling in my head. Something is a little bit different. I've been able to talk quickly lately. My powers of speech have improved. I've been able to work better. I've been funnier. I've been charged. I actually talked to my birth father about this elevated state. He is a Doctor. I also researched manic depression because it feels like I'm in a manic stage. Full of joy most of the time. My curiosity is fueling this passion.

I'm still trying to figure out what it all means. Yesterday, I noticed a beautiful purple flower on a walk. I googled it, and it's called Shooting Star. While lying in bed this morning, getting into alpha brain wave… I saw a dark figure… it woke me up but did not really scare me. I then saw a massive shooting star out the window. That was really cool. The synchronicities are all pointing me to the next level of consciousness. There are many ways to get there, but the Silva mind control came up as a synchronicity a week ago. Also, very important synchronicity: Esther Hicks channelling Abraham. These are the teachings that The Secret was based on. I did manifest that $5 bill. That happened. I did manifest a dog. That happened. The owls and the quail. I jumped out of bed, and the fire alarm beeped at the exact time. According to my medium reading with Peggy, the first thing she received from the other side was that *I am an anomaly*. Anomaly is defined as something that deviates from what is standard, normal, or expected. Maybe our lot being named Fantasia by the realtor was not a coincidence.

June 2, 2023 – Journal Entry

Life continues to be incredible. I'm happy all the time. I've got a list of things that I'm excited to do all the time. The goals on my wall have come true.

We went camping at Ellison with the entire family. It was the best camping trip ever. My entire family agreed. On the first morning, I woke up at 4:20 am and went for a walk while the entire campground slept.

On my walk, there was an educational sign about woodpeckers. One of them was a Lewis woodpecker. Just after reading this, I spotted a red-headed woodpecker that flew right in front of me, and I started to follow it as it moved from tree to tree. It landed in a tree off the path, so I walked to it with the hope of getting a video. I then came across a small memorial that someone set up right near the woodpecker tree. This was a hidden memorial with a little totem pole and many other important items memorializing somebody's loved one. Hidden. Nobody would come across this because the terrain to get to it was filled with dead branches, fallen trees and bushes. This was definitely a sign. The woodpecker led me to this memorial. I have now decided to build a memorial for my spiritual team in the hills above our house. I have ordered four plastic sheet holders. I have found the perfect spot. Right by the location where John and I saw the owl.

I get a feeling that this world is more connected to the other world. Synchronicities are all the time still. Yesterday, on a walk, I was thinking about Barry and listening to music, and I pointed to a tree right next to me. Right at that moment, a woodpecker flew up to me and went right into the tree, exactly where I was pointing. I don't know why I pointed at the tree. It was like something took over me. I did not know the woodpecker was on its way to the tree. Something like that could be almost miraculous, but it did not affect me that much. Stuff like that is happening all the time. I am loving life. I am an anomaly.

I prayed this morning. Out loud. The higher intelligence has been OK with people praying to God. That is just the name of the entity that has created or helps create. I'm not sure. However, this higher intelligence is pulling strings. Or is this a simulation, and as you get closer to what the simulation wants you to do, it pays you back with synchronicities? Kind of like a game of warmer, warmer… now you're hot. Honestly, I'm not sure who I'm praying to. I definitely think my team is involved with my synchronicities. My team is here with me. It's a matter of where I take it. It looks like money is headed my way. My work is going extremely well. My goal is to get it running without me to a certain extent. When it has enough momentum… I could step back. I could focus on whatever comes before me. I've really enjoyed my work my whole life but I'm open to anything the universe presents for me.

Something that helps others. I guess my business helps others. It provides money to people across Canada. It supports my employees. If you can manifest reality… that must be a function

Red Pill in the Universal Matrix

of this world. Are we in a simulation? Probably. I don't know. It's funny that The Matrix was my favourite movie.

June 4, 2022 – Journal Entry

A massive rainbow landed on our house. While sitting on our deck, a beautiful owl flew over our deck. I had my back to the owl, but Lindsay said it flew right toward us and then swooped up right behind me. The next morning, because of a series of messages someone on Twitter was sending me, I decided to go to church. The Twitter person told me that somebody would talk to me when I visited a church. She was right; the priest approached me after the service, recognizing a new face in his flock. He asked me to email him, so I did. I sent him an email informing him about UFOs and the Phenomenon, and I told him, he could contact me if he had any questions. Just like when I decided to be a researcher at university, I am acting like I'm an expert on the subject. Am I actually going to manifest a job related to the Phenomenon? I'm following the manifesting rule about acting like my desired reality is already here. Awesome.

June 7, 2022 – Journal Entry

Yesterday, I went for a morning run up the hill before work. I meditated. Really good. On the way back, the sun was shining, and I saw a purple flower; I took a picture and sent it to Peggy. Minutes later, I see an owl. This reminded me of my walk at Ellison campsite when I saw the grave memorial that the woodpecker took me to. On that walk, I sat down on the cliff edge, saw a purple flower next to me and sent a picture of the flower to Peggy. Moments later, I saw an owl. Perhaps my Dad wants me to connect with Peggy again. Perhaps the universe does.

June 14, 2022 – Journal Entry

Went on a walk with John on Sunday morning. On our walk, I told John that I think the endgame of the UFO stuff is to open the minds of humans. To allow humans to be open to a new realm of possibility. Esther Hicks channels a collective of higher energy entities. They are able to communicate very easily through Esther. I bought the book a couple of months ago, immediately after both Peggy and Andrea recommended it. The book is essentially a transcription of the higher intelligence being fed directly to Esther Hicks - directions related to manifestation; if you believe we are interacting with a higher intelligence, and I 100% do, then this is the book I should read. It's like a bible, except it is written by a modern-day higher intelligence. Wait a second, isn't that the exact backstory of the bible? Cool. So, I shared this new direction with John. Much to my synchronistic surprise, it turns out that John's Dad was given the visualization/manifestation secrets from the higher intelligence his Dad interacted with 40 years ago. It's kind of the secret of this earth. Higher intelligence wants humans to know this secret. If more people truly accept this as truth… it would lead to a better world. It's just a matter of breaking the walls down and opening up minds enough to accept that higher intelligence could speak through a human. I am an "anomaly" who, through exposure to synchronicities and deep research into the UFO phenomenon, has had my eyes open enough to accept

Red Pill in the Universal Matrix

this possibility. Once you accept what is being conveyed as truth…. the world is amazing. In the near future, when I read the book, I will attempt to manifest many things. Why the hell not? I can do anything within the realm of the possible. I suspect the realm of the impossible is not achievable. If my manifestations are good for society, they will definitely be helped out by the Earth game.

June 26, 2022 – Journal Entry

On Friday evening, we went to a party, and the host brought out a giant jug of water. One of the attendees and I got into a disagreement about how to describe the 'jug.' I wanted to call it a carafe, and he wanted to call it a "vessel." I exclaimed. I had never heard the word vessel to describe a water jug before. We dominated the party's conversation with our momentary, meaningless banter.

When I came home, I randomly turned on a movie with Melissa McCarthy, and in one of the first scenes, she used the word "drinking vessel" to describe three shots of tequila. This seemed odd to me, and it stood out as a coincidence.

On Saturday morning, I woke up at exactly 4:20 am. Then I went for a walk with Andrea at 8 am. It turns out that Andrea, the girl I helped in Earth Science 11, is a life-long medium connected with higher intelligence. Higher intelligence communicates directly with her pretty much her entire life. Her life-long spiritual path is extensive. We were Facebook friends, and we have interacted a

Red Pill in the Universal Matrix

bit since high school. When I started to learn about the UFOs, I started posting stuff on Facebook. Andrea, who has a tremendous history of spiritual awakening, could recognize that I was starting to wake up. When I broadcast the quail living on my deck on Facebook live every morning for a week, Andrea knew something was up. We started to chat casually through Facebook Messenger. Right when I'm getting into that level of discovery with my learning, the universe provides me with a friend with direct experience. First John and Peggy, and now Andrea.

On our walk, Andrea recommended a book: "Sacred Contracts" by Caroline Myss. When I started listening to the book, the author used the word 'vessel' about 30 times in the first chapter. The word Vessel became a synchronicity for me in a span of 24 hours; it really grabbed my attention and made me focus on the content of the book. Here is the excerpt from the first chapter:

"I want you to imagine you and me, I'm your Angel, I've got you on a cloud, and I want to talk to you for a minute, and I'm going to say here is the vastness of your spirit. I'm going to give you yet another opportunity to incarnate. What would you like to be? How do you want to become? Not just *be*, put the word *become* in its place. What do you want to learn? Not just learn in terms of spelling, reading and writing, how do you want to divinely absorb the very process of creation you are going to be a part of? A **vessel** of the flow of divine thought into form. This is what life is - it's the experience of becoming a **vessel** of divine thought into form. It's an experience of creation. How do you want to **vessel** that force? That's exactly the language I want you to think. You are going to **vessel** the force of creation. Now that is a great big, huge visualization, and you are going to take that visualization, and you're going to think, how do I want a **vessel** to join creation in such a way and here's how you want to think. You want to think in such a way that it serves the whole creative evolution of humanity."

So, the word vessel comes to me from 3 different sources in a span of 24 hours. That made me take note.

After my walk with Andrea, I played golf with some friends and then I went to Lindsay's sister's wedding anniversary party. At a certain point at the party, I felt like I needed to check my phone to take a video cos it was a beautiful moment. I looked at my phone and it was 4:20 pm.

Right after that, Amanda came up to me, took me aside and told me that a few months back, just like me, the colour red had become an important colour to Amanda. She just loved it. The exact same as me. She came to the party that day wearing bright red, exactly like I did. Both Amanda and I developed a love for the colour red at the same time in our lives. That is weird. 4:20 came twice in one day. Big day. Just don't exactly know why yet.

July 1, 2022 – Journal Entry

I think I might have found the connection between the colour red and Amanda and the day of 420. I went golfing today at Vernon Golf. One of the members of our foursome had a phenomenal round. His putting was phenomenal. Draining 50-foot putts on back-to-back holes. At a certain point, I started to say he was being controlled by a higher power. The weird thing was that he was having back pains, something he had not had before. I vocalized that he was being controlled by a higher power.

I came home and put on the first show that looked interesting to me. I think I was directed to put on that show: Episode 4 of "Surviving Death" on Netflix.

The first story is about a lady who asks her best friend to come back to her as a 'cardinal' after death. The **red** cardinal comes back in a big way. Lands on her shoulder in her front yard and won't leave her.

The next is a story about a lady who asks for **red** balloons as a sign from a loved one. The **red** balloons appear outside her apartment window within a day, hooked on a tree. This is the same red activation story as me. I had asked Tylen for **red** balloons to appear, and the strange affection and guidance from the color red began.

The next story in this episode tells of a man whose son dies; soon after the funeral, he has a voice whisper in his ear… 'I am **Red**.' A week later, a couriered package arrived at his front door. It was a painted picture from a student's parent (his wife is a teacher). It was a picture of a soul-like ghost colored **red**. The person who sent the picture indicated she was compelled to buy it and send it to them. Did not understand why. She bought a weird picture of a **red** soul-like person and sent it to their kid's teacher. It's

Red Pill in the Universal Matrix

definitely a big coincidence when coupled with the husband getting a ghost whisper in his ear… "I am red."

I shared all this information with Amanda at our RED party on July 1. It turns out, Amanda had communication with her deceased brother when he first died, but she was mad and confused and super sad. She could have shut him out. My feeling is that the red is his way of breaking his way back to her. I told Amanda to watch the Netflix show and I refer Amanda to Peggy.

Peggy has a connection to the other side, and I'm certain Amanda's twin brother would want to reconnect with her. I hope she has a session with Peggy cos this feels like the end goal of all the red.

On the day I sent Peggy's email to Amanda, the red balloon I asked for, the origin of my love for red… finally manifested. It was tied to a tree at the end of a driveway on my street.

After connecting with Amanda about red last weekend, I changed our Canada Day party to a red theme. I purchased red umbrellas. I talked about red. I love red. I bought red chairs. I bought a non-alcoholic six-pack of beer called "Red" (without consciously realizing the beer's name was Red). In my emailed invitation to everyone about our Funtastic red-themed party, I said it would be the best party ever. I think it came close.

The northern lights were out big time that night, right over Vernon. They were not quite visible from our pool deck. However, if we would have seen them, it would have been the best party ever. It was already close to the best. It was perfect. All day long, the clouds rolled in and burnt up right before covering our sun. We had sun all day, surrounded by stormy clouds.

Tylen, sleeping at a buddy's house, saw his first owl. Sydney, while sleeping at a friend's house, was compelled to go outside right before bed. She was crying when she saw the northern lights. It was like she was compelled to go outside. Tylen saw the northern lights, too.

> I LOVE MY LIFE. THANK YOU UNIVERSE. PLEASE KEEP ME POINTED IN THE RIGHT DIRECTION TO ACHIEVE ALL MY GOALS. THANK YOU THANK YOU THANK YOU.

Things are manifesting in rapid fire.

My business is absolutely skyrocketing right now. Best quarter ever. Next quarter will be even better. Jim Carrey wrote a cheque to himself for $10 million. He made it happen and then continued to roll in cash. I see that happening to me. Abundance is on its way. My Spiritual team, Dad, Mom, Russ, Barry and whoever else has a hand in this miracle are protecting me, guiding me, guiding and protecting our family. The google description of the angel number 420 number is exactly me. It fits me quite accurately right now:

> "Angel Number 420 is a highly spiritual number that is **connected to the Divine realm and your Guardian Angels**. It is a sign that you are on the right path in your life and that you are making positive changes. The number 420 numerology also carries the energies of hard work, determination, and inner wisdom."

July 4, 2022 – Journal Entry

I just re-read my journal from the past couple of months, confirming the dates and occurrences that happened to me the day I made my appointment with Peggy and the appearance of the wooden spoon, Maureen, and Trish the quail. That is a miraculous story. It is 4:30 am right now. I woke up at 4:20 am again. Last evening, I awoke from my sleep two times to look over at my angel numbers on the clock: 2:04 am and 4:02 am. My emailed message to Amanda this morning:

My Angel number is 420. I was woken up two times last evening by 'My Angels' to look at the clock to see my numbers: 2:04 am and 2:40 am. I wake up. I look, I go back to sleep. On the day we discovered our similar affection for the colour red at the wedding anniversary party, I was compelled to get my phone and shoot a video at exactly 4:20 pm. I also woke up at 4:20 am. My question is, did you watch episode 4 of Surviving Death? If not, are you not ready to accept this potential reality? Now I'm full-out pestering you, and I don't care. "I AM RED."

July 5, 2022 – Journal Entry

Just another minor miracle. Amanda remembered yesterday that her deceased twin brother's favorite color was **red.** He wore **red,** every day. Everybody wore **red** to his funeral. She had blocked out that fact from her mind but it came back yesterday. That is so weird she blocked that out.

It feels like mini miracles are happening all around me.

Dear Spirit Guides: I like it when people laugh. I love being in situations where I and the people I'm with are having a fun time with lots of laughter. If you can help me create situations like this, it would be much appreciated. Thank you so much for everything you have done for me. I feel like you are guiding me and my family to higher levels of happiness. THANK YOU.

Summary Amanda synchronicities related to the color red:

Amanda and I both started loving the color red at the same time even though we live in different cities and we had not seen each other for over a year. We discovered this new shared passion for red when we both wore red to a party. A few days later, I randomly watched a Netflix show that focused on how deceased loved ones come back to connect with living relatives, with each of the 3 connections focusing on the color red. I tell Amanda to watch the show. Amanda remembers that her deceased twin brother's favorite color was red and everybody wore red to his funeral. Amanda makes an appointment with Peggy and connects with her brother.

MUFON - UFO Convention

When my passion for studying UFOs started, my life started to change. It was like I was living in a bit of a dream world. I noticed I had more energy. I was waking up early, ready to go. Ready to take on every day. With a list of audiobooks on my phone and printed books, I spent most of my spare time learning. When you are very interested in something, passion can fill you with energy. It appears I found a big passion.

I joined MUFON – The Mutual UFO Network. MUFON is a US-based non-profit organization composed of civilian volunteers who study reported UFO sightings. It is one of the oldest and largest organizations of its kind, with over 4,000 members worldwide with chapters and representatives in more than 43 countries and all 50 states.

After checking in with Lindsay, I signed up to attend the annual conference on July 7, 2022, in Denver, Colorado. I flew to Denver solo for the weekend. It was an incredible weekend.

July 7, 2022 – To Denver – Journal Entry

> Woke up at exactly 4:20 am - Of course. Flew to Vancouver. Sat beside a retired nurse from Newfoundland. The last thing she said to me was, you have to visit Newfoundland. Exactly the same instructions that were given to me by a person I met at a party a few weeks before. I guess I have to go to Newfoundland, where my birth mother was born.
>
> In the Vancouver airport, I was calm and happy. Flew to Denver. It was a beautiful sunny night. Rented a car and drove to the hotel. Got

a little lost negotiating the one-way streets of downtown Denver and ended up following right behind a bike parade. I checked in at the hotel. My room was in a tower across the street from the check-in area at the hotel. It took me about 10 minutes to get to my room. When I got there, my key card did not work.

Another 15-minute round trip to the front desk to get a functioning key. Finally, I got in my room. I decided to buy some weed and groceries to keep in my room for the weekend. Google mapped a weed place. It said 4 minutes to get there, but I guess that was driving time. I started walking to Weed Place and walked past the Colorado State Parliament buildings.

Encountered a tame bunny on the lawn of the parliament. Videoed and took pictures. Decided to buy a pizza at the place right next to the weed place. It took at least a 25-minute walk to the weed place. Got ID'd. Need a passport to buy weed in Colorado! Got a bootlegger guy to buy a joint. Did not anticipate needing a bootlegger at 48 years old… but it worked out perfectly. He was at the door coming in when I exited the store. Nice guy. Went back and got my pizza. Went to a small grocery store across the street. Stocked up on snacks for the weekend. Started walking back to the hotel. I ate half my pizza on a quiet street, sitting on a cement garden box. I walked back past the parliament buildings.

Took more pictures of myself and the parliament. Got to an intersection and made a decision not to walk past a bunch of homeless people. Why am I going into such detail about the first night?

Because the timing of my arrival back at the hotel became pretty important...

About a minute later, as I was approaching our hotel, I noticed a bright light in the sky making a quick movement. It's not a normal movement. A very high-speed jut, back and forth in the sky and then it stopped.

I instantly went for my phone and started videoing the object. It was a UFO, right above the hotel. I was very excited. My assumption was that the hotel was loaded with UFO people, and this UFO was something they would see all the time. I got about a 5-minute video with the UFO immediately above me, and then it slowly moved out of my line of sight. I quickly walked up the road and it came back into my view. Got another 48-second video of the same orb.

As far as I know, nobody else in Denver videotaped that UFO. I arrived at the UFO conference, and I was the only person who saw and videotaped a UFO above the hotel. Miraculous. Synchronistic. Phenomenal.

I went back to my hotel room, dropped off my groceries, and then went back down to the city street. I wanted to keep looking at the sky. I asked a lady outside having a smoke for a light. We get into a deep conversion. By the end of it, she said, I have to go back inside cos you are freaking me out a bit. This was my first lesson in the way some people react to somebody discussing UFOs. Back in the hotel room, I texted Syd, Brooklyn and Lindsay about my sighting.

Thus begins an absolutely amazing weekend. AMAZING. My path that weekend was directed by the Phenomenon. I kept on being put in front of and connecting with the speakers and organizers and people the Universe wanted me to talk to. It was amazing. The Phenomenon has control over people. It's incredible when the Phenomenon wants to show you a good time…a good time is coming your way. PHENOMENONAL.

July 8, 2022 – First day of conference – Journal Entry

Get up and get a ticket for the Peterson Air Force Base bus tour. On the bus, I start talking with those around me. They end up becoming my all-weekend friends. One guy with a beard sat behind me on the bus, and we chatted. We will call him Beard Guy. The bearded guy was smart and personable.

When I was in the elevator going down to the 2nd floor, I started talking to a calm, smart and soothing lady. She was so calm and emotionally helpful. Throughout the weekend, I would constantly sit down and see her beside me, randomly. A few times, she ended up saying things to me that made perfect sense at exactly the right moment. I enjoyed her company, and I gave her a hug and a thank you on the last day.

After meeting me in the elevator, she decided to go on the Air Force bus tour as well. When I got on the bus, she ended up sitting beside me in the same row, across the aisle. Behind me was Beard Guy. And then, beside the soothing lady sat an older, knowledgeable dude who does not use a phone. He just reads books. Sometimes, he is a bit of a grump, but he was a nice guy and he was interested in what I had to say on the bus and throughout the weekend. We will call him Oscar (the grouch).

The Air Force base tour was great. I shared my video with others, and everybody was very interested. When we got back to the hotel, I watched the tail end of a presentation on the Phoenix Lights. I then went out to the main street of downtown Denver. No car traffic, just a pedestrian street. I walked up the street, and I had this immense feeling of positivity. I feel like I can do good with every interaction and in every situation. I ended up talking with street performers, giving them $5 tips. I paid homeless people when they were polite, especially if they were wearing red. I wore all red at the conference every day.

Came back to the hotel sitting area and proceeded to chat with a lady from New York. She knew very little about the UFO topic. Then I talked to a dude who sat beside me, and he talked about sacred geometry. 369 and the miracles of a fractal-based universe. I then walked to the water cooler, and a guy was standing there and handed me a filled glass. We started to talk and instantly bonded. I then looked at his name tag, and his last name was Hynek. Son of the first head of the USA UFO program in the 1950s and 60s (J. Allen Hynek). I was randomly talking to the Sunday morning keynote speaker. I was starstruck. I got a selfie with him.

Other speakers came up to us while we were talking. I walked with Hynek into the banquet hall. At this point, Oscar the grouch came up to me and he actually had reserved a seat for me at his table.

Oscar made sure I sat with them. Once again, I sat right beside the soothing lady. Some of the people at the table personally knew Grant Cameron. Another guy, a life-long experiencer and his wife became a smoking buddy throughout the weekend. He had the experience of being directly under the massive craft that flew over Phoenix in the 1990's. We had some great chats.

After the keynote speech that night, I went to my room and then decided to go to the hotel bar. I saw a group of conference people, and I walked near their tables, but there were no seats. So I went to the bar. The guy on the bus, beard-guy, was sitting at this table. He must have seen me and came and got me from the bar and invited me back to the table. I sat at the only seat available between 2 grandmas. We chatted. I charmed. At one point, the red-haired grandma lady on my right said to me, do you know who I am? I did not. But it turns out I was sitting beside the President of MUFON and his wife. Another keynote speaker magically appeared in my path. Got a selfie and a hug. Awesome.

The next morning, I get up and go to the 'experiencers' meeting. I sit down randomly, and I'm right beside a soothing lady again. Hundreds of people are at this conference, and I keep randomly, not intentionally, sitting beside the soothing lady. I actually stole somebody's seat who must have left for the bathroom, and the seat beside the soothing lady was the only one open. I did not see her until after I had sat down. Like an AA meeting, people were sharing their personal experiences. A very high-strung couple shared. I felt compelled to connect with them after the group. We bonded. They were very connected to messages being received from some sort of intelligence. However, not all their messages were positive. Some were demonic. I ended up exchanging emails and had to tell her I could not accept that her beliefs were real. I hope I helped her. She indicated that I did help her.

I spoke to Paola Harris for at least an hour. She wrote a book with Jacque Vallee. I spoke with a guy who turned out to be the afternoon speaker. I ended up going to dinner with him. Every turn I made, I talked to someone important and highly connected. My path felt so carefully laid out. One of the things that surprised me was that I had a deeper knowledge of the topic than a lot of the people I spoke to. I was up to date on the most recent occurrences in the disclosure efforts. I had read more than most people I interacted with.

Got to be one of the most exciting weekends ever. Finding my passion... absolutely.

======================

This was the last entry I made in my journal. My life continued to be ladened with synchronicities and positivity... I'm not sure why I stopped my journal entries; I guess I felt I had better things to do with my time than writing stuff in a journal.

It's hard for me to explain how directed I felt my path was at the MUFON conference. Every time I went somewhere, every time I turned around, I ran into and bonded with someone who put me face to face with a speaker, author or someone with a tremendous involvement with the UFO topic. Being the only person who filmed a UAP at the conference facilitated this. Many people wanted to see my video. I submitted the video to MUFON,

Red Pill in the Universal Matrix

and a few weeks later, it was confirmed by their video people that I had captured an actual UFO. I knew that the instant I saw it. The quick motion it made. Not a normal object. There is no rational explanation for that orb of light.

Why was I so lucky to see and film the UFO? I've come to realize that there are no coincidences in this amazing reality we live in. Why me? Not sure. But if I had to guess…I am active on social media. I had a TikTok addiction. I am active on #ufotwitter. I believe the Phenomenon has a goal to open people's minds. Making people believe something else beyond what we have been force-fed by school and, government and media. I was a perfect candidate to spread the message. I own my own company. I can't be fired for posting my views on social media. I have family and friends that love me and they are not going to abandon me if I start voicing views that don't fit the norm. Maybe I was the most effective person at the conference for the Phenomenon to present. Maybe the Phenomenon could predict, back then, that I was someone who would end up writing a book. Opening minds. For someone with as big of passion as I have on the topic, me seeing and filming a UFO on the first night of the UFO conference… now that is a synchronicity.

Little did I know the experience at the UFO conference would start a chain reaction of learning that continues to this day. It's like my higher self has been prepping me for this series of events my entire life.

I flew home from Denver, and I had a layover at the Vancouver airport. I sat down in the holding area about 1 hour before my flight took off. Someone called my name, and I looked up and I saw one of my daughter's best friends. Their school trip was coming home from a European vacation, and they happened to be on my flight.

When I boarded the plane and got to my seat, another one of my daughter's school friends was sitting beside me. She asked if she could slide over and take my window seat. I agreed and I took her aisle seat. I then see another friend coming down the aisle of the plane. She happens to sit right beside me, across the aisle.

I did not know this about her prior, but she is very open-minded, and we talked about UFOs and higher intelligence for the entire flight back home. Coincidence? No, just an extension of what I felt was happening to me the entire weekend in Denver. My path is guided. There are no coincidences.

Family Camping Trip –
2 days after the UFO Convention

I got home from Denver with a new appreciation for the reality that we live in. A few days after arriving home, our family left on our annual camping trip. Every year, our entire family meets in a small community a few hours from our home. My wife's three sisters and their families join us. Each family has three kids. We circle up our motorhomes and trailers and relax for a week. We spend the week soaking up the sun on the beach of a very beautiful lake. Grandma comes. Other friends join us. It is literally better than a Hawaiian vacation in nature with our entire family. This year was different. This year was better.

On the first night of our vacation, my wife noticed that our neighbours from back home were also camping close to us. At this point, I was starting to believe that there is no such thing as coincidences. I went and met our neighbors and spoke to them for about an hour until I heard Grandma calling my name to come back to our campsite.

When I returned to our campsite, we had our first campfire and everybody was sitting around as the daylight was slowly leaving. I sat down, and on the horizon I saw a very bright light come up from behind the mountains across the lake and slowly start moving toward us. I pretty much instantly recognized it as a UFO. I scrambled back to our motorhome and got my phone to video it. My family all saw it. At first, my brother-in-law's started to say it was a plane. I knew it was the same type of light that I had videoed in Denver a few nights before. It was a classic orb. The light slowly moved across the sky and then did a right angle turn and slowly started moving

Red Pill in the Universal Matrix

back across the lake. I videoed it all the way across the lake until it disappeared on the other side of the lake. I was very excited. It was surreal. Whatever it was, it appeared to have followed me home from Denver.

I returned to the campfire and sat down. I got my glasses on. I would sit away from the fire a bit so my view of the sky was less affected by the firelight. I must admit, in this early stage of my awakening to this new reality, I was pretty addicted to the night sky. The night went on and I saw an unusual amount of shooting stars. That was cool.

Eventually, around 11 pm, everybody went to bed. I was still pretty excited so I went and sat on a community picnic table that was close to our homestead. I had a few hoots of a joint, which was my first indulgence of the day. I was looking at the sky and I asked the sky for another presentation of the Phenomenon.

Within 5 seconds of asking, another orb appeared in the exact area of the sky where I was looking. It slowly came up from behind a mountain and very slowly travelled directly over top of me. I was videoing the entire time. While I was videoing, some local residents who were down at the beach also saw the orb.

One of them started to yell, "Take me home!". At that point, I did not think that was a very smart thing to be yelling. The light travelled in a random path, not really a straight line and ended up going over the lake and down behind the mountain on the other side of the lake. It was visible in the sky for about 6 minutes.

I decided to get more video footage, so I went to meet up with the people on the beach who also saw the UFO. As I approached them, as an icebreaker, I told them I was with the Men in Black. They chuckled and stated, "I plead the fifth." I then proceeded to interview them with my camera rolling. They didn't like that I was videoing them, but they wanted to share their story. Apparently, last year, they witnessed a plane flying over the lake with a UFO buzzing around the plane. They also described seeing an object earlier that day. They had talked about it but did not know what it was. I thought it was awesome that I had other witnesses who acknowledged the existence of the orb of light that could not be explained.

When they left, I went back to my neighbours campsite; they were still awake. But this time, I was pretty excited, and I must have come across as pretty crazy to my neighbors. I didn't really care, though. While talking to them, we saw another light come up from behind the mountain across the lake. I videoed it. I posted most of these videos on my Instagram account.

I then proceeded back to my motorhome and sat outside my motorhome, looking up at the sky. Another UAP went clearly across the sky. It was probably 11 am when I decided to go to bed. That night,, while lying in bed, I did actually feel some nervousness. At that point, I did not know if I was dealing with aliens or what I was dealing with. I had read enough about alien abductions to realize that the experience of being abducted can be pretty fearful, at least the first time you are abducted. When I closed my eyes, I had a vision of almost demonic-like entities coming into the beginning of my dream state. I had read that some people pray to Jesus to avoid bad stuff. I did that. I also prayed a little to my spiritual team, my Mom, Dad, Barry and Russ.

Eventually, I got to sleep but woke up a few hours later, still pretty excited. I got out of the motorhome and walked down to the beach about 5 am. As the sun was coming up, I saw a family of ducks coming toward me. A mom and four babies. As they approached, I realized it was not a duck; it was a merganser. To me, this was very exciting. Lindsay's Dad, Russ, used to always get excited when he saw mergansers. Russ would always shout, "It's a goddam merganser!" Every time, like it was the first time he saw one. I followed the merganser family down the beach that morning, and eventually, they swam across the lake.

The merganser family took my anxiety away. I felt like Russ and my spiritual team were with me. I sat down on the beach again and laid back. Closed my eyes and fell asleep as the morning sun was starting to warm things up. I was awoken by something splashing in the water. The family of mergansers had come back and was about 10 feet from me. I felt joy. I thanked my spiritual team.

When I returned to the family that morning, I was very excited to share my videos of the merganser family. Russ loved camping. He would have loved to be with us and the mergansers made us feel he was.

That day, the whole group sat down at the beach, about 100 feet from our homestead of campers. We started to notice an unusual amount of butterflies everywhere. It was awesome. Later that day, one of the kids ventured away from our beach location and found what must have been a butterfly mating area. Literally, hundreds of butterflies swarming and landing on the banks of the lake. The butterflies flew around us on the beach all week. It was amazing.

This week at camping was a continuation of my trip to Denver. I'm literally high on life. I'm not sure what it all means, but I'm happier than

I've ever been. I'm feeling spiritually connected to my loved ones. I feel like they are with me, with us.

One day, a majestic bald eagle was flying across the lake. I was standing in the lake watching it when it turned ninety degrees and flew right across the lake directly at our family at the beach. The huge bald eagle then landed in the tree right above where we were sitting at the beach. It stayed in the tree for hours. At one point, two black ravens started to swoop and attack the bald eagle, but it held its ground. We all felt Russ was with us, in that amazing bird, spending the day with his entire family.

The second night, I perched myself a little bit back from the fire, looking intently at the sky. Again, I saw many shooting stars, not like the shooting stars I had seen throughout my entire life. These were pure streaks of light. No burning chunks coming off as a meteor burns in Earth's atmosphere. I felt the number of shooting stars that I saw was considerably higher than normal.

Moreover, they came to the exact locations where I was looking at the sky. It was questionable. But then something happened that was completely unexplainable. I was looking straight above me. A shooting star came into my line of sight from behind a tree and then stopped immediately above me. It disappeared and then reappeared instantaneously and continued to shoot across the sky.

When it disappeared momentarily, it shifted position in the sky by about 12 inches in my line of sight, like the meteor made a left turn for a bit and then continued in the original direction. That was unexplainable. But it was a clue given to me by whatever is running this reality.

Red Pill in the Universal Matrix

The re-directed shooting star and the number of crystal-clear shooting stars made me question the night sky. I'm somebody who has had a lifelong interest in shooting stars. I've planned camping trips around the Pleiades meteor shower for multiple years. I've let my young kids stay up as late as they could to watch for shooting stars. I'm familiar with the frequency of shooting stars during a meteor shower. I know what meteors look like. On this camping trip, the meteors came too frequently and were too clean (void or any burning chunks). What am I suggesting? At the time, I knew something was different, but I was happy to see so many shooting stars. As more experiences were put in my path, I now believe that the night sky is like a computer screen, controllable by something.

Every night, orbs would appear, and I would film them. My family members would spot them and send me chasing them with my camera. Sometimes, the path of the orbs would take them behind trees, so I would have to follow them down the road or across the parking lot. My family started to joke: "There goes Cale!" We all saw the orbs, but nobody was as interested in them as I was.

My kids and I started to say earlier in the year that the Phenomenon was helping our family be happy. Creating the best situations. Our lives will be elevated in 2022. This trip was no exception.

One day on the trip, the ladies in our group went on their annual mom float. It used to be just the Moms that would escape for the day but this year, our daughters were old enough to join the Mom float. Floatation devices are attached together with coolers in tow and the ladies set out on the lake to get out of the line of sight of Dads and the remaining younger kids. The Dads stay back at the beach and make sure all the kids have sunscreen, naps, and other parenting requirements. The ladies stay away for as long as they want.

Sometimes, requests are relayed to bring them more booze, and the cooler gets replenished via a jet ski trip. This year, the ladies were out on the float when the water started getting a little choppy, so the mom float got anchored to some large poles that were in the lake, around the corner from our beach, out of sight from the little kids.

As 'luck' would have it, a local resident happened to be travelling by on the maiden voyage of his houseboat converted into a party barge, and through a series of drunken cat calls issued by the ladies, the houseboat owner, named Shameen invited the crew of inebriated ladies aboard the party barge. Shameen just happened to be testing the ability of his houseboat to move with the newly built floating dance floor.

Shameen was accompanied by an 18-year-old male companion, Conner, who helped Shameen build the party barge. Our ladies had been on their mom's float for a couple of hours when the party barge happened, and their relaxation state was in top form - they were in the mood to party. No more sitting on floaties and dingy on the wavy lake. Now, they had a houseboat with an accompanying dance barge.

Music was cranked, and a dance party ensued. Conner and Shameen had happened upon a bit of heaven, and ladies felt the same way. The mom float lasted all afternoon, and when the moms eventually floated back to our beach, they were ecstatic, pronouncing the best mom's float in the past 15 years.

Shameen and Conner were invited back to our homestead that evening. When they arrived, I happened to be walking by and I instantly knew these were the gentlemen who had hosted our wives and daughters. I instantly could feel they were good people.

Genuine people. I welcomed them into our campground and made them feel as welcome as possible. They added a local component to our trip. That night Shameen took us down to the beach and introduced me and my daughters to locals having a fire and small party at the beach. It was awesome; we got a chance to meet many very open-minded people.

Throughout the trip we would interact with our newfound group of local friends. At one point, Shameen came to the beach with his two baby goats and geese. They were tame. The young kids had their own personal petting zoo arrive our beach. Phenomenal.

An annual event that the Dads do each year rivalling the Mom float, is to pack up a vehicle and head to the local golf course. We pack enough booze to make sure all Dads can drink a beer each hole. We play nine holes, so by the end of the round, not a fuck is given. Somehow, many years ago, we formed teams for the annual golf event. We play a 'best-ball' format. My two competitive hockey background brothers-in-law, Cody and Brad, form one team, and whoever else is with us that year forms the other team.

For the past 15 years, whatever team we have assembled has never been able to beat Cody and Brad. This year, for the first time, our 14-year-old sons, Tylen and Rylie, were invited to come with us. In the state of positivity I had been in, I felt like this would be the year we would topple

Red Pill in the Universal Matrix

Brad and Cody's mountain of victories. My internal state of joy and positivity was so elevated.

On the way to the course, I turned down the music and I announced to the combatants that this would be the year that Cody and Brad would be taught a lesson. As the game proceeded, our team managed to put the needed shots up at the right times, and we won the first five holes out of a possible 9, and the decisive victory was ours. First time in 15 years, phenomenal.

This whole trip, I felt like I was living in a dreamland of elevated happiness. Thankful that my reality was being steered to positive happenings. This was very much bolstered by the fact that every night, I got to experience UFOs, a topic I had been obsessively learning about for the past six months.

After the first night of multiple UFOs, I did have a little bit of fear of abduction. I had read books that described abduction experiences in detail. I was aware of the possibility. Fortunately, I had just spent the weekend at the MUFON convention, surrounded by people who had experience working with people who had interacted with Phenomenon. I sent a private message to a lady who seemed well-connected to the Phenomenon on the second day of our trip. Here is my message:

Hi Linda,

Last evening, camping with my family, I was able to videotape three more orbs similar to the one above the Denver Sheraton. The Phenomenon is presenting itself to me. The second orb pretty much appeared right after I asked for it. Didn't get much sleep last night. I'm not sure exactly what

Red Pill in the Universal Matrix

I'm supposed to do. But it appears the Phenomenon has something in mind for me.

Linda's response: *Just keep documenting and pay attention. Never approach one.*

That was good enough for me. The small bit of fear that I felt on night one of the camping trip did not return. I felt bolstered by my spiritual team. I was so fearless that there were several nights on the trip where I would lie in the dark on a picnic table near the beach, away from campers or lights, and everybody was asleep. I fell asleep a few times, looking up at the stars.

The fear that I felt that first-night camping did not come back until one night a few months later when we saw a UFO so close that I felt I could hit it with a golf ball. If I was going to get abducted, it would have happened that night… but we will get to that later.

Upon returning to Vernon in the middle of July, it was like I was living in a dream. I was so happy. My family was happy. The people we interacted with were happy. The weather was always perfect. Business was growing. I now had a passion, or as my wife felt, an obsession with the night sky. I would go for walks around dusk. I set up a circle of chairs up the mountain behind our house. I envisioned a night where I would go with a small group of open-minded people, and we would call for a presentation of the Phenomenon. I never actually did that because it wasn't necessary.

The Phenomenon continued to present itself throughout the summer. I would sit out on the patio beds at night and wait for UAPs. I filmed many. I put some of the videos on Twitter, TikTok and Instagram. Our house has a nice view and I can see most of the sky in every direction. People that

Red Pill in the Universal Matrix

saw the UAPs with us, started having their own presentations. They would send me their videos.

My friend Red and his wife were outside gardening on a sunny Sunday afternoon when Red saw a metallic orb slowly travelling across the sky. He filmed it. It was an amazing UAP sighting. Metallic objects slowly move across the sky. We had a similar sighting during the daytime at our house.

My wife saw the silver metallic object first. We were outside on a sunny weekend afternoon when she saw the metallic object travel above some powerline near our house. I had time to get my phone and video it. The object slowly travelled up the mountainside and then did a right turn and travelled all the way across our backyard, following the skyline until it went over the mountain and out of site. Daytime sightings were awesome. Mind opening.

In August, my daughters Sydney and Brooklyn went on a camping road trip with 2 of their friends. The four teenagers set out on an adventure to find an isolated spot on a lake about 1 hour from our home. That night, they had a special presentation of the Phenomenon. Something I had witnessed above our home in Vernon about one week prior.

A repeating light appears in the sky and travels quickly across the sky in a random path. The light appears from nothing, travels like a slow shooting star for about 2 seconds and then disappears. Immediately after it disappears, a new light manifests in the same starting point as the first light and repeats the same path. This repeats for about a minute, with probably about 40 lights appearing and disappearing at the same point in the sky.

Each light is only in the sky for about 2 seconds. Just like the orbs that hover in the sky for several minutes, there is no astrological explanation for this light pattern.

When the girls came home from camping, and Sydney described these lights to me, they matched exactly what I had seen one week earlier above our house. I believe the Phenomenon has a bag of tricks it uses to open people's minds. This repeating light trick is a good one. It's not too shocking. It is not fear-provoking. It is simply something you can't explain especially if you have any background in studying the night sky. Mind opening.

One night during the summer, John, the basketball coach and his wife came over to our house for drinks. It was a beautiful night. Whilst conversing in our pool, we heard a loud explosion sound. We got out of the pool and went to the edge of the yard, which has a better view of the city below. We then saw a huge explosion at the electrical station at the bottom of our hill.

The booming sound of the explosion followed a few seconds after seeing it. Our power went out. It was quite interesting to see the explosion and it added to the intrigue of the evening. Fortunately, I happened to have recently charged our bluetooth speaker, and we continued to socialize. We adjourned to our balcony and continued the festivities as the sun went down. It was a great night. When it got dark, a large bright orb appeared in the sky and slowly made its way toward our house. I, of course, videoed the orb. This was a period of my life when I was highly charged by things happening in the sky. We spoke about the light as it was slowly moving overhead.

The light made a ninety-degree turn and headed east. I explained to John that I had seen many of these lights in the past few weeks. I told him that if it followed the same pattern as the other lights, it would eventually fade out of view. That's what it did. From the brightest object in the night sky, it vanished into nothing.

I went golfing in the summer with three good friends at the Vernon Golf and Country Club. It was a beautiful day. We were teeing off on the 7th hole when something appeared in the sky I had never seen before and have not seen since.

Emanating near a lone cloud in the clear sky appeared what I can only equate to metallic birds. Only you could not distinguish any wings on the objects. The objects flew through the sky and then disappeared. Other objects would appear and then disappear. I pointed out the objects to my friends. We all stood there looking up at something that could not be explained. It was incredible.

As I was standing on the tee-off box at the time (it was my turn to shoot), I did not return to my golf bag to get my phone. I really regretted that decision as I have not seen a similar presentation of the Phenomenon since that day. It was incredible. It was also the first time 2 of my golf buddies had seen anything that could not be explained. Even for me, those lights were emotionally moving. The disappearing metallic birds lasted for about 30 seconds before they all vanished. I told my friends it was a presentation of the Phenomenon. I told them that strange happenings such as this have been happening to me quite a bit. My friends did not want to talk about it. There was a strange uncomfortable feeling for me and my golf cart mate as we drove away from the tee-off box on the 7th hole. I did not press about the topic because, half the time, I feel people think I'm a bit crazy, and they simply do not want to talk about anything that does not fit into the scientific explanation of reality.

A few holes later, I asked my golf cart mate if he had seen the videos on my Instagram account. His response was that there are alternative rational explanations for my videos. Fair enough.

Everybody will open their minds to new possibilities in their own time. I have learned not to try and force my views on others. When people want to talk about it with me, they will bring up the subject. I will share my views. No need to force my views on others. It took me a while to figure that out. I had several people think I'm a bit crazy in the past year. Fortunately, this doesn't bother me.

Night of the Shooting Stars

Another memorable night during the summer occurred in August. We had a small party at our house with about 7 couples. By this time, I had posted several videos on my Instagram page. I was also the only person posting articles about UFOs on my Facebook feed. I'm still the only person out of 400+ Facebook friends to openly post information about UFOs. I can post a picture of my kids or some other 'normal' happenings in my life on my Facebook page, and I will have dozens of people that will like or comment on my pictures. Facebook posts about UFOs did not get much, if any, interaction from my friends or family. It's understandable, most people do not want to be associated with the tinfoil hat stigma that has been broadcast by the governments and media for the last 70+ years.

The night of the party, we were standing on our front deck and everybody started seeing shooting stars. It was cool. I wasn't buying it. I explained to everybody that the shooting stars we saw were too clean. Too perfect. Crystal clear with no evidence of anything burning, as is the case when a meteor burns up in the earth's atmosphere. It was at this moment, with every partygoer looking up at the sky, a huge meteor burnt all the way across the sky, leaving a tail of burning pieces scattering off the main meteor. Now that was what a shooting star is supposed to look like. Everybody was in awe of the biggest meteor they had ever seen. Phenomenal.

There were orbs that night. They would rise above a distant mountain, circle over our city and return back to the mountain they originated from. I videoed some of them, but frankly, it was rude of me to be videoing while entertaining guests.

Red Pill in the Universal Matrix

One guest proclaimed, "That's a plane." Fair enough, if you take a quick look at a light in the sky and your mind is closed to the possibility of something else…it could be perceived as a plane. I believe people will have their minds opened to something other than nuts and bolts reality soon enough.

Something happened that night that was a huge clue to me in relation to the nature of this reality. My daughter Sydney has always been a great person to listen to me as I'm trying to figure out what is going on. Many times she has told me, now that sounds crazy. But she is open-minded. She doesn't close her mind to the amazing possibilities of this reality. At one point during the party that night, Sydney joined us on the balcony. We were all looking at the sky whilst talking. Sydney and I were leaning over the railing, looking at the sky when Sydney stated, "Look at that!" She then described the repeating light that she saw while camping with Brooklyn and their 2 friends. The lights started just above the horizon and zipped across the sky horizontally. When one would vanish, a new one would start out. Sydney described the location of the lights very clearly to me, as they were close to the horizon and we had identifiable markers on the mountains where the lights started and where they stopped. I couldn't see the lights she was seeing. About 30 seconds later, they stopped. I never saw them. We then talked about the lights and made absolutely sure I was looking in the right spots in the sky. I was. About 20 minutes later, Lindsay had joined our conversation and then Sydney saw the lights again, in the exact same spot, exhibiting the same start and stop characteristics. This time, Lindsay confirmed she could see them as well. I could not see them. I'm not blind, and at that point in my life, I was pretty obsessed with seeing anything I could in the night sky. I could see the stars crystal clear. I could not see the lights that were being presented to Sydney and Lindsay. It was an interesting happening. The Phenomenon was able to present something selectively to the consciousness of some people, but not others. It provided me with a clue about the universal matrix that we live in. I was grateful.

Red Pill in the Universal Matrix

People With Supernatural Experiences
Coming Out Of The Woodwork

One of the interesting things that occurred when I started broadcasting my beliefs about UFOs and the Phenomenon to those around me, I became a bit of a lightning rod for people with supernatural occurrences in their background. Most people don't want to talk about strange happenings in their own life because people think they're crazy, or perhaps they don't want to think about stuff that they can't explain.

As soon as I started posting stuff about UFOs and talking about UFOs, people saw me as someone with a very open mind to weird stuff. On the night of the shooting stars party, one of our friends told a story about how she and her friends saw a metallic UFO fly immediately overhead in the middle of the day when they were teenagers in Lumby. Saw it clear as day. She is open-minded.

Another one of the party attendees described how she had an out-of-body experience in her past. I pointed her in the direction of remote viewing. Another attendee at the party shared with me that he grew up in a home with a ghost. Doors slamming right in front of him, objects moving, voices. Ghosts. It turns out I have 3 close friends, university graduates, that have interacted with ghosts their entire lives. To this day. These are rational, intelligent people who have incorporated supernatural occurrences into their belief structure, and miracles manifest regularly. We had another friend who met a baby bigfoot when she was a kid. She has had interactions with aliens. She gets quite anxious if the topic of aliens is brought up because she believes that will bring them to her – something she wants to avoid.

Apparently, I have been surrounded by people my whole life who have experienced the supernatural. I was late to the supernatural game, but when I started broadcasting my belief of UFOs on Facebook, the supernatural believers had someone to talk to. Someone who would have an open mind. Needless to say, it was a great party.

At another social gathering, one of the ladies who I had just met told me how she saw a huge creature fly out of her back yard a few months earlier. She described this creature as almost like a small dragon or a pterodactyl dinosaur. This wasn't the first time she had seen this creature. I did some research, and she is not alone. Over the past several decades, there have been several documented sightings with the exact same descriptions of pterodactyl creatures. Just like bigfoot or other supernatural occurrences, I believe the Phenomenon is going into overdrive, trying to open people's minds to something different.

At yet another social gathering, someone I just met told me about the lead singer of a local band who had a UFO disk land in the field right by their farm, in Armstrong, in the middle of the day. He witnessed actual beings emerge from the craft and then get back in and fly away. Obviously this changed his life. Another high school friend, told me a story about how he was at the local Kalamalka Lake view point with his mother. A UFO hovered pretty much right above them. An actual silver craft in the middle of the day. When he notified his mother about the craft, she looked at it and then walked away. She wanted nothing to do with that craft. It was a pretty incredible experience, you won't forget something like that.

My friend Red was open-minded about UAPs. He recognized how passionate I was and appreciates anyone with a passion. The Phenomenon generated a presentation for him and his wife. He even was able to video the silver UFO in the daytime. But then Red, perhaps, allowed his mind to close off a bit.

On the same night that Red told me he was thinking about writing a book, Red told me about a very strange occurrence that started happening in his basement. The door to his cold storage room in his basement kept on opening up. Red would close the door securely and the next day, it would be open again. His family did not open the door.

Either somebody is breaking into their house each night, or …. a ghost is opening the door. My interpretation is that Red's higher self wants him to have his mind open to the amazing reality that we live in. Opening minds… that is a goal of the Phenomenon.

Red Pill in the Universal Matrix

Asking the Sky for a Sign

After coming back from the camping trip, I spent many nights out looking at the sky. Sometimes I would ask the sky for a presentation from the Phenomenon. Sometimes I would ask my spiritual team. I felt my spiritual team was and is always with me. So when I asked the sky for a sign, I guess I was talking to them. On several occasions, when asking, I had the sky answer. The first time I was standing on my deck at home, in the exact position I was looking, was an incredibly bright flash. It was brighter than several stars combined, almost like a massive camera flash in the exact area of the sky I was looking at.

A few weeks later, it happened again. This time I was on a night walk in the hills above my home. Next, it happened towards the end of the summer when I took my son and his cousin on a downhill biking trip to a nearby ski hill. I walked up the hill to get away from the lights of the village. I was waiting for a UFO to appear. I asked the sky for a presentation of the Phenomenon, and instantly, the huge camera flashed in the sky. I was grateful.

The next time it happened, I was on a walk above my house looking at an orb. I wasn't videoing it. Then the sky flashed right by the orb, and I instantly started videoing it. These sky flashes gave me further insight as to what this reality is. There is no natural explanation for this. It really makes me feel like the sky is like a computer screen, completely controlled by something.

In 2024, Sydney and I were on our deck at home, looking at 2 small orbs travelling across the sky.

A bright flash occurred right beside the orbs, and Sydney said, "Did you see that?" Yes, I did. Sydney said that was the third time she had seen a flash like that. I told her I'd seen flashes several times, but it was the first time somebody else had seen the same burst of light. Both of us witnessed the unexplainable flash of light. Also in 2024, Peggy told me that she had witnessed a similar flash of light in the night's sky. I feel that if you reach a certain level of open-mindedness in the Earth game, the game can show you various anomalies in the sky.

Roots and Blues Festival

One of the most incredible presentations of the Phenomenon happened at the Roots and Blues Festival in Salmon Arm, BC. This is an annual music festival attended by thousands of people. The night we went, Tom Cochrane was playing. We made some plans with some friends to park our motorhomes in a nearby parking lot in the middle of town so that after the concert we could sleep over. We got to the concert, and there was an amazing rainbow. The concert was awesome. You could feel the positivity in the crowd.

After Tom Cochrane finished, we walked back to our motorhomes. My wife, her sister, my friend, and I stood around the motorhome at the end of the night, chatting about the night's events and listening to the band that was still playing back at the festival. My wife's sister, Jill, stated, "What is that?!" She pointed up, and the 4 of us looked up at something that was completely unexplainable. Right over the top of us were 3 lights forming a triangle.

The lights moved together, and slowly crept over us silently. I instantly scrambled for my phone, but by the time I got it out, the object had moved out of our line of sight. It was, by far, the closest UFO I had ever seen. It was not a single orb, like all the other UFOs that we had seen. The object gave the perception of being a solid craft with three lights on the corner of the triangle.

My friend went to bed right away in his motorhome. I don't think he wanted anything to do with whatever we saw. Lindsay, Jill, and I went into our motorhome. I was charged up. Sleep did not come easy for me that night. To me, this UAP put me into a new category.

Again, the thought of abduction became a consideration. If I was attracting an actual craft and not just bright orbs in the sky, that was a different ball game. I still had a strong faith that my spiritual team was always with me. If abduction is in the cards, I have faith that all will work out for the better. Eventually, my small bit of nervousness dissipated.

Upon further reflection, the lights were most likely a slightly elevated presentation of the Phenomenon. No craft just lights organized to look like a craft. If I were to bet, that is what we saw. Mind opening... absolutely.

My Team

As I have been going through this incredible period of my life, I have had a strong belief that my parents, Lindsay's Dad, Russ, and my God-father Barry, have been helping our family. Essentially, we are pulling strings, making adjustments, and just making sure our family is doing OK. It's kind of like the movie, The Adjustment Bureau. I pray to my Team on occasion. I thank them. I feel they are with me all the time.

Originally, I felt owls were my father's doing. My mother became the quail. I began to associate the woodpecker with Barry, and Russ was bald eagles and God damn mergansers. But then owls started appearing in situations that I did not associate with my Dad. My connection to this group of deceased loved ones became "My Team."

I created a Spotify playlist with the songs I most associate with my Team. The weird thing is, besides my father, none of these people have a memorial or grave site. Given their importance to me and the love I feel for them, I decided to create a memorial for them close to my home. I went on several walks in the forest above my house, searching for the perfect spot. I did not want a location where random people would accidentally walk by.

Eventually, I found the location, away from any path, at the edge of a hidden meadow on the mountain. It was close to the spot where John and I had a fairly significant owl encounter at the exact moment I brought up Lindsay's Dad in our conversation.

Red Pill in the Universal Matrix

During my first visit to this meadow, I identified the perfect tree. A few weeks later, I went back with a weed whacker to cut a path through the tall grass in the meadow to get to the tree. There was an owl sitting in the tree. That was a great sign. I ordered plastic page protectors and created 4 individual picture collages for each loved one. It took me about a month. I also built a stand to house the 4 framed monuments.

One day, Lindsay and the kids went to visit Grandma at the farm, and I decided to stay home to finish my memorial display. It was made of wood. It was a hot Saturday afternoon. I started the walk to my location with the stand on my back because it was the easiest way to carry it. It takes about 25 minutes to walk to the memorial tree location from my house.

When I was halfway to the location, an owl flew out of a nearby tree in the exact direction I was going. As I continued down the path, the same owl flew out of another tree. The owl followed me all the way to the side of the meadow. It was fitting. It was amazing, and I know my loved ones were with me every step of that day. I attached the memorial to the tree. I was listening to my playlist making me feel the strong emotions of love I feel for my Team. It was an amazing day.

Since creating this memorial, I have taken several walks to that tree. It has become a special location, and several amazing animal occurrences have taken place in the meadow adjacent to the tree. One day a hawk came and landed on the actual tree and proceeded to swoop down at me many times. Upon leaving that day, the hawk stayed with me as I walked home. Surreal. Of course, I videoed the hawk's many swoops at me and posted the video.

Red Pill in the Universal Matrix

Another day, I stopped in the field and looked up at the sky, and at that exact moment, a hummingbird flew exactly where I was looking, about 3 feet above me, and stopped, hovering for about 5 seconds.

Another day, a dragonfly flew around me for at least 15 minutes until I had to go home. Another day, walking back from the site, I am not sure what prompted me to do this, but I pointed up at a random tree on my path, and at that exact moment, a woodpecker that I had not seen, flew into the tree. Thank you, Barry.

Red Pill in the Universal Matrix

Owls of 2022

As I have explained, early in my sobriety, owls played a very important role in maintaining my faith that my Dad was supporting my efforts to quit drinking. After the first couple of years, I had completely learned my lesson, sober for life, and the thought of drinking again simply does not exist for me anymore. The unusual number of owls manifesting in my life dissipated. Until 2022. The live owls started appearing to me and our family at an incredible frequency. I saw five owls the same week as Father's Day. In August, I had 4 beautiful owl feathers come across my path as I was walking.

One feather in particular stood out as amazing. I was walking in the woods, and there was a red ribbon tied to a tree. I was drawn to the red ribbon. I walked towards it. The ribbon was tied to a branch above my head. I walked underneath the ribbon and looked up.

On a branch directly above the ribbon was a single amazing, beautiful owl feather, just caught on a branch. You better believe that made me feel good. We went over to Lindsay's sister's house one night for a visit. The next morning, there was an owl feather on the patio outside of their kitchen.

One night, we sat on our patio with some friends, and an owl flew right toward us. It swooped by our deck and over our house. It went and sat in a tree in our backyard.

One night we had an owl sitting in a tree right in front of our yard. We were all admiring it when my son Tylen called me from a friend's house,

Red Pill in the Universal Matrix

and an owl was sitting on the chain link fence right beside the playground where he and his buddy were hanging out.

One night, I heard an owl hoot, and I went out by our pool to see if I could spot it. I did not see it, but it was sitting on the back of one of our pool chairs, and it flew right by me. That scared the heck out of me. I actually requested my Team not to do that again. One night an owl flew right into our backyard and was hopping on our grass. One night an owl landed on the top of our house, and I was outside filming the owl when an orb flew over. That was awesome.

One night, I was driving down the road, and I saw something under a street light up ahead. I slowed down because I thought it was a cat. When I got close, I was happy to see it was an owl. Sitting in the middle of the road, looking right at me. I came to a stop about 20 feet from the Owl. He just stood there for about 20 seconds and then flew away. The exact same thing happened to my daughter Sydney as she and her friends were driving. The owls were perched in the middle of the road.

When I was driving Tylen to the golf course one day, an owl swooped right in front of our car. About 2 minutes later, another owl flew out and flew right beside our car. 2 owls on 1 trip on the 5-minute drive to Hillview golf course.

My daughter Brooklyn had multiple weeks where she has seen 5 or more owls. They just appear in our path. We love them.

When I took Sydney to her first basketball tryout at the University, Brooklyn came to meet me at the gym. But she texted me from outside the gym to let me know there was an owl sitting on top of the gym. As

Red Pill in the Universal Matrix

Brooklyn has been walking to and from school, there have been 3 owls sitting in a tree right along her path. When she worked at Sparkling Hill Resort, she would see owls almost every night.

Just last week, Brooklyn came home from university, and a big owl sat in a tree in front of our house. She announced this is like the 6th owl I have seen this week. Lately, owls tend to appear more when all the kids are home.

The re-emergence of owls at this period of my life is amazing. To me, the owls are no longer a message of support for quitting drinking. My belief is now that owls are manifesting to show we are on the right path. Right as I started to have this realization…a very weird thing happened. In my Facebook feed, a random advertisement appeared for a Spotify podcast. The podcast was about how to quit drinking.

The advertisement had a completely red background, and the host of the podcast was Dave Lewis. That's my Dad's name. Synchronicity? Coincidence? I truly believe my Dad's intelligence is still alive in some reality.

Red Dragonfly

One morning, Andrea came over and we went for a walk and had a deep conversation. After she left, I went behind our house to digest some of the information she had shared with me. I stood in the open hillside listening to meditation music and noticed a red dragonfly hovering around me. I notice things that are red.

Later that week, I went golfing and on the first hole, I noticed another red dragonfly. All through the golf round, I kept on seeing red dragonflies. Next week, different course, more red dragonflies. From that point forward, in 2022, every time I went golfing, I had red dragonfly with me. This is not mind-blowing, but I was appreciative. I love the colour red.

Putting the Right People in Your Path

One thing I have come to learn is that this reality can put the right people in your path at the right time. Some would say that the frequency you are emitting from inside of you manifests in your 3D reality. Until my spiritual awakening in 2022, I did not know how many people in my life lived with different aspects of the supernatural interacting in their lives But as my learning progressed, the exact people I needed came into my life.

As I was reading books and learning, I was eager to share my knowledge with those around me. So much so, that I eventually had to make a rule for myself: do not talk about UFOs unless people ask me about them. Initially, it was a difficult rule to follow. I was passionate about the topic.

Several times, I saw people's facial expressions change as I brought up the subject. People would politely excuse themselves from the conversation. I developed defence mechanisms. I'd say things like, that's what I've been reading about anyway, or "Stick that in your country song." And then I would change the subject.

John

John, our basketball coach was the perfect person to have come into my path, just as I was diving deep into the subject. The information available in books really is quite incredible. Mind-blowing. My passion for the topic needed to be discussed with somebody open-minded. It's good to be able to talk with someone who has an open mind. John grew up in a family that was frequented by UFOs and supernatural occurrences. He had extensive, deep, direct experiences with what I was reading about. We started going for long hikes where we would compare notes and try to figure out exactly what was going on. It's all a huge mystery, but this reality is offering so many clues.

Peggy

Peggy, our lifelong friend, no longer seemed fraudulent to me. Peggy is somebody who can connect with the intelligences that have crossed over to the other side. It was a gift the universe gave us to be friends with Peggy. In the summer, Peggy was at our house with her kids for an afternoon swim. She was standing in the middle of our pool, and a bird flew over and landed on her shoulder.

A few years later, another bird landed on Peggy. My interpretation, the universe likes Peggy. She is light. My sessions with Peggy have been nothing short of miraculous. The information she conveyed to me after doing her readings was incredible.

In my 2 sessions with Peggy, the information provided to her from the other side was congruent with my understanding of reality at that time and gave me pretty much exactly the information I needed to hear. It cemented a belief that the intelligence that populated my parent's Earth avatars is still in existence, somehow in another part of this reality. Do I believe they are in heaven? No. I believe their intelligence lives on as a small component of the quantum computer simulating this reality. Stick that in your country song.

Andrea

I've always had a strong interest in astronomy. When I was 6 years old, my parents bought me an expensive telescope. My Dad and I would set it up outside and focus on various objects. In high school, for one of my grade 11 electives, I took earth science because there was an astronomy component in the yearlong course. I was already taking physics and chemistry so I did not need another science to get into university. I could have taken woodwork or some other fun elective, but I chose to follow my interest in astronomy. It was in this class that I met Andrea. Andrea was attractive, and my perception was that she hung out with the 'popular' group in high school. That was my 16-year-old evaluation of her. I helped Andrea with some earth science assignments. It was a brief interaction, but Andrea became an important part of my path in 2022. What I've come to learn is that this reality can put the right people in your path when you need them.

Andrea is perhaps the most spiritually awake person I know personally. Our paths have crossed a few times in the past 3 decades, but I was not aware of her level of knowledge about the great possibilities available to us in this amazing reality. As I started to post information about UFOs on Facebook, Andrea and I connected. To me, she appeared open minded about the subject. I asked her to go for a hike to chat. She agreed. As we started talking, Andrea had great insight about my path and gave me great advice and shared some over her own experiences. I would experience synchronicities about the books Andrea recommended. It was very useful to hear messaging from Andrea that I needed to, "slow down."

Peggys' connection to the other side also vocalized this slow down messaging. It was helpful. Andrea had a direct connection to a higher intelligence. Beyond the incredible abilities associated with a psychic medium. Kind of like my own personal Esther Hicks that I can talk to in real life. Reality bends around Andrea. I think she should write her own book. We went for about 4 walks. After each walk, I would need time to digest the information and guidance she gave me.

One night, after one of our walks, Andrea and I ended up on our front deck at home, chatting with Lindsay and my daughter Brooklyn. Andrea was in the process of manifesting a business where she could help kids. Andrea is a talented therapist. She had thought of a name for the business, the Robin Hood foundation. She would provide counselling and therapy groups for paying adults, allowing her to help the kids for free. Andrea knows one of the rules of this reality, if your passions are aligned with doing good for other people, you will be more successful. It was an enjoyable evening.

The next day, my family left to go camping for the weekend. We were returning to the campground where we had seen the multitude of UFO's about a month earlier. When everyone went to sleep, I returned to the picnic table, the darkest area, allowing me an excellent panoramic view of the entire sky. I lay on my back on top of a picnic table. I had my earphones in, listening to a random Spotify playlist. I eventually fell asleep. I must have been asleep for at least half an hour when all of a sudden, I was startled awake. Almost as if something had turned up the volume on my air pods. The song that was playing was the Disney theme song from Robin Hood.

Robin Hood and Little John, walking through the forest,
Laughing back and forth at what the other'n has to say,
Reminiscing this and that and having such a good time,
Oo-de-lally, oo-de-lally, golly, what a day

Red Pill in the Universal Matrix

I had not heard the song since I was a kid. I had not downloaded the song. It was really kind of spooky that we were talking about Robin Hood the night before. Take from the rich, give to the poor. I'm not sure how that song ended up in my playlist. I listen to country music. I don't listen to nursery rhymes or Disney theme songs.

We had an incredible weekend. We ended up getting invited on to a houseboat rented by a number of people from the local community. They were celebrating 3 birthdays. It was awesome. On the drive home, my mind started to wonder about the synchronicity inherent in the Robin Hood song coming through on my headphones to wake me up. I then realized that the giving theme portrayed in the classic Robin Hood tale is congruent with the directions about giving back described in the book The Secret. There is an entire chapter dedicated to giving back. Make donations. Help others. What you put out to the universe comes back to you. Just as I was putting this together, 2 bright red vehicles came around the corner and zoomed by us. A cherry red corvette and a new red pickup truck. On this highway, you can travel for periods of 30 minutes or more and not see another vehicle. The 2 bright red vehicles appearing in conjunction with my thinking about the contemplation of the Robin Hood synchronicity cemented my belief that my life will be better if I give back. Help others. Donate to charities that help others. I've started paying homeless people. I've made donations to local charities that help homeless people. This is a complete change of character for me.

I grew up in a household that was very 'frugal'. My mother would cut coupons and travel to different grocery stores to purchase the least expensive items. We would not go out for meals... such a waste of money. We did not go on vacations. Hotels... are a complete waste of money. I remember the first time I got straight A's in grade 9. We decided that we would go out to dinner to celebrate. My mom ordered water and said she would just pick food off our plates because she was not hungry. This angered my Dad. We ended up leaving the restaurant because the argument that ensued was not going to get solved prior to meals arriving. So much for celebrating my straight-A report card. My mom kind of won that argument because we did not waste money on a meal out. My mother was not cheap, she just really did not like wasting money. As I was starting out living on my own, I was very frugal, just like my mom. When Lindsay and I first moved out together, I used to add up every penny that we spent together and everything was divided 50/50. Later, when Lindsay's sisters moved in with us, we divided the bills equally, right down to the penny. That's just the way I was. That frugalness slowly eroded as we started to make money.

When I read 'The Secret,' there was a chapter devoted to giving back. Charitable donations and helping others get paid back by the Universe. It's a rule of this amazing reality. When I first learned this, I tested it. Being charitable to others was really kind of against my lifelong beliefs. But this year has really changed my lifelong beliefs. The test I did was on a Sunday morning golf outing with some friends. We usually will play some sort of skins match or other monetary incentive on the golf match to add extra fun to the game. Usually, the golfer with the least skins pays for a beverage of the other golfers. That morning, I played great, and I was the clear winner. Me and my 2 golf buddies enjoyed breakfast on the clubhouse patio. I was feeling amazing. Given the new knowledge about the universe paying you back and probably the first time I ever done this, I went inside the clubhouse and told the waitress I would pay for the bill. It cost me about

$44. It felt good, and my friends were surprised and appreciative. The next Sunday, I went golfing with 2 other friends. When I arrived at the course that morning, one of my golf friends emerged from the pro shop and announced, "I got you, Lewis; golf is on me this morning." This was a completely altruistic gesture from this friend. This is the first time ever that one of my friends has paid for my golf round. These were different friends than the previous Sunday. The kicker is the cost of the 9-hole golf round, and the shared cart is $44+tax. It was awesome. Give to others, and the universe pays you back.

Vegas Trip. 444.

In September of 2022, myself and 12 Dads from the "Tuesday Night Club" went on a weekend trip to Las Vegas. Before Covid, we would go on a fun trip every year, it had been a few years since we were able to go away. We left on a Thursday morning, and we got to the airport at about 4:30 am. I checked in and decided to go to Tim Hortons to get some breakfast and coffee. When I sat down to take out my phone, I noticed it was 4:44 am. Interesting. We flew to Vegas and got down to our hotel pool as soon as we could.

Spent the afternoon at the pool and then returned to our rooms to get ready for the night's shenanigans. I did not take my phone to the pool so when I returned to the room, I picked my phone and it was exactly 4:44pm. Interesting. As the trip progressed, the number 44 kept on coming up in my reality. It was a new angel number. It kept on coming up. From that point forward, to this day, I see 444 and 44 everywhere. And I mean everywhere. I seem to look at the time at the 44th minute all day long.

When I'm on the treadmill, I will look to see my stats and it will be the 44th second or the 144 calories burned. It's incredible. When the 44's started appearing to me, one Friday, I posted it on twitter in the morning. That night we attended a Halloween bon fire at Lindsay's sister's house. I dressed as 'red' man. As the party was winding down, I looked down at the fire to see the logs in the fire formed a perfect 4.

A few days later when I was driving by my wife's school, I noticed the Christmas lights in the trees in front of the school formed 444, one 4 in each tree. A friend who I told about the occurrence of 4's in my life had a

Red Pill in the Universal Matrix

bucket in his back yard and when he picked up the bucket, hundreds of ants under the bucket formed a perfect 4. He took a picture and sent it to me. I've posted all these occurrences of 444 on twitter.

There was a husband and wife team of mediums from Australia that came through on my Reels feed in Instagram. I commented on one of her posts and she reached out to me and indicated that she had received messaging about me from the source feeding her information that I would be contacting her that day. She told me I was one of the 144,000 light workers or 'starseeds.'

At the time, I did not really know what she was talking about but then videos started coming in my feeds about what light workers are. I guess I could be one of those. I'm willing to share anything I've come to believe to be true to anyone that is interested. I have had a track record of opening people's minds to something beyond a nuts and bolts reality. I think that is part of what a light worker does.

But back to Vegas… we had a blast. After the lulls of Covid, it was great to be able to travel with my buddies again. On the first full day of our trip, I went down to the pool and reserved our poolside location for our group. As I was soaking up the sun, poolside, I started to chat with the couple that was in the chair beside me. Pleasant conversation.

Eventually, I learned that he was a navy pilot. He actually works at a school that teaches pilots to fly. His job was equivalent to the character Maverick played by Tom Cruise in Top Gun 2. Interesting. I gingerly shared my interest in UAP's and recounted some of my knowledge about the flight characteristics of the wingless crafts. I then asked him if he had

Red Pill in the Universal Matrix

ever saw a UAP. He thought about it for a second and then said he was actually not supposed to talk about it but…. he had 4 separate encounters with tic tac UAP's while flying. He said it scared the shit out of him. He said that as a pilot of some of the most expensive, fastest jets in the world, you want to be the top dog in the air. You have faith that in a dog fight, your craft would be able to outmaneuver the enemy. He said the UAP's flew by his airplane like he wasn't even moving. They were ridiculously faster than his plane. That scared him.

I find it incredible that universe put this gentleman in my path. I suspect I would be one of the only people around who would be as interested and knowledgeable about military interactions with UAP's and I just happen to sit down beside a Top Gun Pilot who has had 4 separate in-flight interactions with these highly advanced crafts. Phenomenal.

Artificial General Intelligence - AGI

One of my passions has been learning about Artificial Intelligence. In about 2012, I read a book by Raymond Kurzweil called "The Singularity is Near". Mr. Kurzweil is a very intelligent person who has invented many things in his life. He is a futurist. He sees where technology is going, and he invents things that become possible when technology catches up to his thinking. Currently, he is the head of engineering at Google. In his book, Kurzweil documents how the advancement of intelligence on Earth is very clearly following an exponential curve. For thousands of years, intelligence has progressed on the flat bottom part of the exponential curve. But then computers entered the picture and things started to change rapidly. Computing speed doubled every 2 years. Computing costs decreased rapidly.

The size of computing power also decreased rapidly. With the advent of quantum computing, the exponential doubling continues. The Singularity is the point where humans give birth to Artificial General Intelligence (AGI). When I read the book, they had conducted a survey with every AI expert they could talk to and 90% of them felt that we would reach AGI by 2050.

With the recent development of ChatGPT, experts in the field of AI are starting to shout that we need to slow down. We need to pause. We need to get a handle on AI safety. The problem is, not everyone is going to slow down. They can't control AGI development in all countries. They can't even control it within their own country. Several incredibly smart people feel that the development of AGI is the single biggest existential threat to humanity. Way more dangerous than nuclear war, a pandemic, an asteroid

Red Pill in the Universal Matrix

or any other possible calamity. Why is it so dangerous? Why can't we just pull the plug on the machine?

The problem lies in the fact that a true AGI system will be smarter than all humans combined. Infinitely smarter. So smart that even our brightest, smartest minds can't begin to scratch the surface of how intelligent AGI will become. We can't fathom it. It will happen quickly in a matter of days. We won't be able to tell it's happening. Just tonight, I saw an interview on 60-minutes with the head of Microsoft. He indicates that their top engineers don't really understand how chatGPT works. How it comes up with its answers. They are trying to figure it out. Back engineering it. Sometimes, they do figure things out, and they make improvements. Elon Musk has been shouting to everyone about the dangers of AI for several years.

Humans have created millions of species extinctions on Earth simply because we are the most intelligent creatures. We don't intend to wipe out species, it just happens as we have goals to achieve and pay little attention to lesser intelligent creatures. Extinction is a side effect. Depending on the motivation of an AGI and what it sees as important to achieve, it is not likely the AGI will take the intelligence of humans as something that needs to be cherished. We will be like ants. Not really something to consider.

This year, I read a book called "Life 3.0" which is a modern-day summary of the status of AI development in the world. I finished the book on a Sunday night and the next morning, ChatGPT was introduced to the masses. Coincidence? Or did my higher self direct me to read the exact right book at the exact right time? I logged in to ChatGPT on that Monday morning and started churning out blog articles for my business.

When my co-workers arrived at work that morning, I had created 5 legitimate articles that could be posted on our company website. It took me about 20 minutes to feed the AI system with the correct prompts.

Artificial General Intelligence is right around the corner.

Currently, the majority of AI experts predict true AGI will be here by 2030. It could be this year. Elon Musk has recently predicted we will reach AGI by 2026. When you get to the elbow of an exponential curve, things progress really fast. We are now at that point. Right now.

The biggest threat to the survival of the human species is happening right now. There really is no way to stop it. The country or the company that develops AGI first will have an unsurmountable advantage. Companies are not going to stop this race. Unfortunately, the finish line could be the end of biological life as we know it.

The Universal Matrix –
The Simulation Hypothesis

In August 2022, I was chilling after work, listening to the most recent installment of the Spotify podcast, "That UFO Podcast". The host was interviewing an author, Rizwan Virk. A graduate of MIT and Stanford, Rizwan Virk is a successful entrepreneur, video game pioneer, film producer, venture capitalist, computer scientist and bestselling author. The podcast discussed his most recent book, "The Simulation Hypothesis."

As I listened to the podcast, my level of excitement elevated considerably. I was getting chills of excitement. I knew I had to read this book. Synchronicities occurred as I listened to that podcast, like I had been preparing my whole life to hear the information discussed. During the podcast, Rizwan referenced books and movies that related to the Simulation Hypothesis and I had already read most of the books and seen the movies. The Matrix was my favourite movie of all time. As I had been experiencing supernatural happenings for the last 6 months, I had been feeling like we could be living in a matrix-like reality. I understood the different aspects of quantum physics that scientifically support the Simulation Hypothesis.

I read The Simulation Hypothesis, and my belief system changed. On Twitter, my posts started to be focused completely about the simulation theory, away from UFOs and the Phenomenon. I now believe 100%, we are living in computer generated simulation.

I had a monumental synchronicity associated with this book. Before the podcast, I had never heard of the Simulation Hypothesis. I felt like we might be living in 'The Matrix' because of all the weird stuff that was happening, but that was the extent of my knowledge on simulation. In the spring of 2022, at our first family camping trip of the season, my wife took a picture of me looking at Okanagan Lake. I'm not sure why I did it, but I raised my hands as if offering to hug the world.

From that point forward, I took many pictures of myself in various locations, with this same pose. I asked my friends and family members to take the same pose in multiple pictures. I took pictures of my shadow on the golf course with the same pose. I did not know why I was doing this; it just felt good. It became a weird thing I was doing. I don't know why.

When I got the book "The Simulation Hypothesis," the cover of the book showed a human-like robot with its arms extended, exactly as I had been doing in my personal pictures for the past 3 months. I then understood why I had been taking pictures with my arms extended.

I have been very fortunate to have been given several personal experiences that support my belief in the Earth Simulation.

1. Synchronicities

I've had the distinct pleasure of experiencing synchronicities. That means reality has been adjusted in strange ways to provide me with mind-blowing co-incidences. I see synchronicities as a clues offered by my higher self, my spiritual team, the Phenomenon, the Universe, the Source, God or the intelligence behind the simulation itself. These could all be the same thing. I don't know who or what creates the synchronicities. I feel like my Dad created the owls in my path. However, a lot of synchronicities occur based on our own thoughts coupled with actual occurrences in real life. I now think the part of me that is situated on the quantum computer, my higher self, can take over my thinking prior to exposure to an owl or some other future occurrence. For synchronicities that run deeper, combining more people, things and situations to send you a message, to say the universe arranged those… I don't have that much faith in a magical universe. I don't have that much faith in God. I see it more likely that my higher self, the component of me with higher access to the simulating engine is creating the synchronicities. My higher self is the player behind my avatar, controlling me in the game of Earth. And it is just a game. Earth is simply an advanced virtual reality game but we will get to that in a bit.

Synchronicities involving putting the exact right people in your path at the exact right time can be downright spooky. John, a lifelong Phenomenon experiencer, just happened to be in the parent's basketball hotel room the night I read the book, "Skinwalkers in the Pentagon." That was a freaking mind-opening book. I was completely amazed at the supernatural occurrences that happened around Skinwalker Ranch. When I shared with the group of parents and coaches in our Vancouver Hotel room that night, everybody must have thought I was a bit crazy. But deep down, John didn't. John became someone I depended on to discuss the miracles of this existence.

When my level of knowledge expanded, Andrea just happened to be waiting in the wings to pick up where John left off. Having first-hand

Red Pill in the Universal Matrix

experiences of the supernatural, primary sources of information to add to my obsessive research, was really good luck. But I don't really believe too much in luck anymore. The simulation will put the right people in your path for whatever lessons you are supposed to learn in this life. Get closer to the path you are supposed to follow, and the synchronicities will start manifesting.

2. Manifestation

Manifestation is real. I was excited and dreamed of owning a home with a fantastic view for years, it manifested considerably quicker than I anticipated. I was obsessively excited about UFOs, and they manifested. I'm not going to try to convince you that manifestation is real. It freaking is. If you don't believe it, you have nothing to lose by testing it. Manifest or pray about something small and see what happens. Imagine a future scenario for yourself and actually feel the emotions as if the scenario has already manifested. Pretend the event has already happened and feel the gratitude. See how long before that scenario manifests in your 3D reality. If it doesn't work, read the book, "The Secret." Google search Esther Hicks and watch some of her videos or read one of her books.

I believe that the consciousness of every player in the game of Earth is connected to the simulating computer. Carl Jung would describe this as the collective unconscious. We create our 3D reality through our collective thoughts. Focusing on the things that make you grateful in your life will manifest more of the things that make you grateful. If an entire country stopped watching the constant stream of negative, divisive, vibration-lowering stories force-fed to us by the media and started practicing gratitude on a regular basis, this country would transform into an incredible place. If the whole world were able to practice gratitude and not focus on the news, the 3D reality would transform into a new amazing world. But that is getting ahead of ourselves. Start with you. Once you change your attitude a bit, it will most likely spread to other family members. An attitude of gratitude is the key. Maybe some friends will want to swallow your new pill of happiness. What you have inside your consciousness, somehow manifests into your 3D reality. Miraculous? Absolutely. You have the capability to create miracles just by visualizing something and feeling emotions like your visualization has already manifested. We live in a simulation. The Simulating computer is all-powerful. The simulating computer likes feelings of gratitude. The higher the feeling of gratitude, the more likely your manifestation happens. Thank goodness. Thank god. Thank the intelligence that created this reality.

3. The Night Sky responding to my Consciousness – The Phenomenon

UFOs were my gateway to awakening. When my beliefs changed, my world started to open up to magical orbs. Standing by myself, looking at the night sky and asking for a presentation of the Phenomenon, resulting in a miraculous orb of light appearing exactly in the sky where I was looking… that made me feel someone or something was hearing me. But not only hearing me but also seeing where I was looking up at the nights sky. This belief was cemented when I would see camera-like flashes, exactly where I was looking in the night sky. Like the sky was answering my request visually. Like having a conversation with this reality. How the fuck could this possibly be happening? I don't believe the orbs I see in the sky are actual material spacecraft. The camera-like flash is not a small explosion of actual matter. The lights and orbs are simply gifts from my higher self, clues about what is possible in this amazing virtual world.

4. Selective presentations of the Phenomenon

One of the biggest clues about the nature of this reality was presentations of the Phenomenon that could be seen by other people, but not by me. When I stood on the front deck with Sydney and Lindsay they could see the orb travelling repeatedly across the horizon but I definitely could not see them, that was extremely useful information. When I stood in the driveway with Nicole in Los Angeles and she could see the triangular craft moving around the top of the constellation Orion and I definitely could not see it, that was another clue. The Phenomenon can interact with the individual consciousness of people and make some things visible to certain people, while not presenting to other witnesses. How the fuck does it do that? Think about it, there are amazing demonstrations of lights in the sky, that are only visible to some observers.

5. Owls and Animals

The number of owls me and my family members have seen is simply not normal. The fact that owls have consistently appeared at the exact moment they have, providing me with messaging to help me along my path is amazing. Having the quail manifest on our front deck at the exact time I felt I was connecting with my mom… amazing. In 2022,

I had so many amazing encounters with animals. Owls, eagles, hawks, hummingbirds, butterflies, dragonflies, praying mantis, bears, coyotes, snakes, skunks, deer and many others would come into my path. I was able to capture some of the amazing animal interactions on video and posted a lot of them on my Instagram. Some of the weirder occurrences included being able to walk right up to deer, cows, or a skunk or when an owl, eagle or hawk would manifest at important times. I came within 10 feet of a bear and a coyote. Butterflies and dragonflies landed on me. While sitting outside, I had a bird land right on my knee. It was a really amazing year for animals. I feel that animals can be used by the Simulation to bolster belief and help us along our path, assuming we are on the right path.

6. Intelligence lives on after death

Read the book, "Signs, the secret language of the Universe" by Laura Lynne Jackson. You will learn that many people received messaging from deceased family members who have crossed to the other side. It's quite common. All you have to do is be open to it. My experiences with Peggy have been miraculous. I did not talk to Peggy prior to our sessions. I did not tell her the questions I wanted answered. But the answers and directions were given to her from the other side.

Another clue offered by this reality is the Near-Death Experiences documented by millions of people. So much information about the nature of this reality can be gleaned from the experiences of near-death survivors. One of the common occurrences of NDE survivors is a full life review. A full review of your entire life, including the time you spent in the womb. A good percentage of near-death experiencers are shown every single occurrence of every waking moment of their lives, presented in perfect clarity, instantly. Time does not exist in this other reality. Your entire stream of consciousness of your Earth life is being recorded. To me, this is nothing other than a very powerful quantum computer with a massive hard drive recording the happenings of every player in the game. I would recommend reading "Dying to Be Me: My Journey from Cancer, to Near Death, to True Healing" by Anita Moorjani.

I'm not alone in my belief in the Universal Matrix. Several genius-level intellects and spiritual leaders agree. When Elon Musk was interviewed on the Lex Friedman podcast, Lex asked Elon, "Assuming we develop Artificial General Intelligence and you could ask the all-knowing computer one question, what would you ask?" Elon gives the question some thought and then responds, "What is outside the simulation?" It's a very good question. In what reality is this super-computer located? Is it on a future Earth or some other planet? I certainly do not believe a bunch of human bodies are being stored in life-sustaining pods, as displayed in the movie "The Matrix." I believe the intelligence (soul) that is being broadcast into every human avatar is being sourced from one incredibly powerful quantum computer. We are all part of the same intelligence. We are one.

One thing is almost certain, in whatever reality that computer is sitting, it is highly **un**likely that reality is more beautiful or wondrous than Earth. The physical beauty of nature and the perfection of Earth is mind-boggling. The simulators really created an amazing planet, and God could be another word for simulating intelligence.

When I read the book, "The Simulation Hypothesis", the book provided a rational explanation for everything supernatural. For the first 48 years of my life, my beliefs were centred on scientific materialism. The supernatural started presenting in my reality in the past couple of years. The Simulation Hypothesis combines observed verified scientific and mathematical facts while providing a perfectly sound explanation of how all the supernatural occurrences in this Earth reality could manifest. One of my lifelong goals has been to understand the nature of reality. I truly believe the Simulation Hypothesis is the explanation I was looking for. To me, it is truth. We live in a Universal Matrix.

Forty years ago, one of the first and most advanced video games was "pong." One ball bounces around the screen. 2 rectangles and a dot. Forty years later, you can put on a virtual reality headset and enjoy an actual game of ping pong with another human player in another city, country or continent. Your virtual game of ping pong is so realistic that you will forget you are not actually playing in the real world. The ping pong player avatars are photo-realistic. The ping pong table and the room you are playing in is indistinguishable from real life. Technology is advancing at such a rapid rate. Virtual reality worlds already exist, combining millions of avatars from around the world in photo-realistic worlds. The technology is getting better every year. Have you ever put on a pair of virtual reality goggles and walked around New York City or any of the other cities that have been 'virtualized'? It is amazing. The technology is that good, in 40 years of advancement. In a few decades, technological advancement will take us to a point where we can enter these virtual worlds without wearing virtual reality goggles. An interface that duplicates the brain signals that create our dreams. Full immersion in a virtual simulation. We will be able to create a simulation that is indistinguishable from real life, with no goggles and no haptic suit. We will be able to create millions of these simulations.

Nick Bostrum, an Oxford professor, postulated the following argument. One of the following 3 propositions must be true:

1) If an intelligent species reaches the advanced technological growth stage that humans have achieved, something will stop the advancement of technology.

OR

(2) All technologically advanced species decide not to create simulations.

OR

(3) We are almost certainly living in a computer simulation.

In other words, unless something stops the advancement of technology, humans will soon be able to create simulations indistinguishable from real life. If one simulation is possible, it will be likely that billions of simulations will be created. The chances of this 3D Earth reality being the 1 base reality is literally 1 in billions. Many believe that we could be in an ancestor simulation, getting a chance to live the last generation before humans evolved into non-biological entities. Some of us got to grow up before the advent of smartphones... ideal, really. Perhaps we also get to witness a true contact moment, where the masses get to witness open interaction with another intelligent species, which will be entertaining.

Quantum Physics provides support for the Simulation Hypothesis. Essentially, small particles are not small particles until a human being observes them. Somehow, human consciousness interacts with and manifests the actual characteristics of the particle. When you study the characteristics of very small particles, it is impossible to predict the location of a particle unless a human observes the particle. Before the observation, the particle exists only as a probability wave.

You might have heard of the Schrodinger's cat analogy. A cat is in a cardboard box. The cat is symbolic of a small particle. We are not sure if the cat in the box is alive or dead. In fact, the cat is both alive and dead at the same time. Equally dead and equally alive indefinitely until a human being opens the box and observes the cat. As soon as a human observes the cat, it manifests as either dead or alive. As soon as human consciousness observes a particle, it jumps out of the probability wave and manifests into an actual particle with specific characteristics. Without human consciousness interacting, reality at the quantum level remains undetermined.

Human consciousness has to interact with our 3D Earth reality in order for physical particles to manifest.

Another weird characteristic of quantum physics is called quantum entanglement. Einstein called this spooky action at a distance. When 2 particles are quantumly entangled, they are instantaneously connected. If you observe the spin of one particle on earth and move another quantum-entangled particle to the edge of our galaxy, light years away, the instant you observe the spin of the Earth-based particle, you will be able to predict with 100% accuracy the spin of the quantum-entangled particle on the other side of the galaxy. When 2 particles are quantum entangled, observing the characteristics of one particle instantly manifests the characteristic of the other particle, regardless of how far apart the particles are. Scientists from Sweden won the 2022 Nobel Prize for physics, proving the spooky characteristics of quantum entanglement. Just think about this: there is no delay between observed particle characteristics. Observing one particle creates instant manifestation in the other particle. If everyone's consciousness is linked to a simulating computer, quantum entanglement would be an ideal characteristic for computing speed.

I apologize for my rudimentary explanation of quantum physics. The Simulation Hypothesis book does an excellent job of explaining why AI, Quantum Physics, and Eastern Mystics all agree we are in a video game.

Mind opening books

As shit started happening to me and I started connecting the dots, following the signs, I asked myself, Why me? Why am I so lucky? Why is this all happening to me? One possible explanation is books. One of my personality characteristics is that I can focus pretty well on whatever I'm doing. I'm driven. When I have an interest in something, I follow it. In some cases, if my interest is strong enough, I will obsessively follow that interest to the point where I must ensure I maintain balance in my life. I thank Lindsay for keeping me balanced. I enjoy learning about stuff I'm interested in. I've always been like that.

For the first half of my life, my reading focused on scientific explanations of reality. I had a pretty good foundation of knowledge and beliefs. But then I learned UFOs interact with military pilots and a whole new world opened for me. I started reading books obsessively and I increased my knowledge of the supernatural. My belief system changed, and the supernatural started to manifest in my life. How come the supernatural does not appear for everyone? I think it has to do with your beliefs. You must reach a certain level in the game. Obviously, there have to be rules for any game. The Earth game must have rules. By reading mind-opening books and believing the information being communicated, I increased my game level. The more I understood, the more our reality shared with me. Here is a list of some of the most mind-opening books and movies that kept me pointed in the right direction:

Artificial Intelligence

Books:

- The Singularity is Near – Ray Kurzweil
- Superintellgence – Nick Bostrom
- Life 3.0 - Max Tegmark

Movies:

- Her – Spike Jonze
- Ex Machina - Alex Garland

UFOs:

Books:

- The Messengers: Owls, Synchronicity and the UFO Abductee - *Mike Clelland*
- Skinwalkers at the Pentagon - *Colm A. Kelleher, George Knapp, and James T. Lacatski*
- American Cosmic - *Diana Walsh Pasulka*
- Operation Trojan Horse – *John Keel*
- Imminent – *Luis Elizondo*

Movies:

- The Phenomenon – *James Fox*

TV:

- Skinwalker Ranch – *History Channel*

Manifestation:

Books:

- The Secret - Rhonda Byrne
- Ask, and it is Given – Esther and Jerry Hicks
- The Law of Attraction – Esther and Jerry Hicks

Red Pill in the Universal Matrix

Simulation:

Books:

- The Simulation Hypothesis – *Rizwan Virk*
- My Big TOE (Theory of Everything) - *Tom Campbell*

Movies:

- The Matrix - *the Wachowskis*
- The Adjustment Bureau – *based on a story by Philip K. Dick*

Jan 16, 2023 – Reading with Peggy

In January 2023, I scheduled another reading from Peggy. I believe Peggy is a conduit for receiving information from my higher self. At the time of the reading, Peggy did not know anything about my beliefs related to the simulation or really anything about the spiritual/intellectual path I was on. Other than the random people on #ufotwitter, nobody really knows about my beliefs because it's a difficult concept for most to fathom. Once again, I did not ask Peggy any questions prior to the reading. The following is what came through to her.

You have grown into the man you were born to be (there is applause). Literally, a whole group of ancestors behind you all clapping, giving you a standing ovation. For some reason, this makes me think of your Birth Dad and his accomplishments in his life. I don't know but there is a tie there somehow.

They are proud of you. Your Mom and Dad are at the forefront of the group, and Barry is beside them. It's like this path, your spiritual part, your evolution in this, was one of the last key aspects for you to grow and evolve into.

Everything is about butterflies for you right now. Transformation. Growth. Expansion.

I definitely feel your Mom (your adopted Mom – Patricia). I am referring to your parents that who adopted you and raised you as your Mom and Dad. They deserve recognition. Just as they honour you now.

There are some interesting ancestral genes from a long time ago that are being presented here (I'm not sure what that means). Your DNA is unique, and it doesn't just come from your birth parents. There is more to it than just that. DNA replication and expansion, have an interesting history. Then I saw an image of you as a little Native boy with a headdress on with a Native elder talking over the fire (past life?).

There are some amazing things in store for you. Amazing experiences ahead! You are ready. In answer to one of your questions, "You are ready." You've harnessed the power of spiritual law, you are smart enough to understand quantum physics, and you are ready to fully expand yourself. It's going to be amazing. A whole new level for you of expansion, dreams, awareness, connection, & interconnectedness. That is a big one for you. You are going to experience things on a whole other level now. Embrace that. Feel that. It's beautiful.

Yes, you are doing what you need to do for your family. Open up. Continue to open up. You are showing the way. It's beautiful.

You are going on a journey; it's going to be life changing – transformational. Like a rocket ship. Fasten your seatbelt and get ready for the ride! "You are called."

What did you always want to be as a child? There is still curiosity and fascination there. Follow your curiosity and see what it leads to.

Have you ever heard of remote viewing? This all ties in somehow. You do have the ability to connect telepathically with intelligent beings, and there is constant communication.

Red Pill in the Universal Matrix

What do you want? Where do you see your greatest growth being this year? The sky is the limit for you – and you know there is no limit – the sky is limitless. Your answers lie in that phrase.

Your Mom acknowledges that you are becoming what you are meant to be. I see her holding out a pan of freshly baked cookies, 12. Yes, the number 12 has significance for you.

Your ancestors from way back are coming through now. Your birth father's grandfather or great-grandfather. He is holding a very old watch. There is significance there to old times – European. I keep feeling a doctor vibe from way down the lineage, but I connected to you. Honestly, whatever you set your mind to, you can achieve. Really, it's all up to you. What you want to create in your life, for yourself and for your family, but don't forget about the part for humanity, being of service, being an open vessel for spirit to work through as well. It's all connected... good job!

Peggy told me she had never received messaging anything close to this before. Never before had the word quantum physics come up in a reading. Coincidentally, I had already read about remote viewing and utilized my Grandpa's golden watch as one of the items I was visualizing as part of the preliminary steps in removing my consciousness from my body. I truly feel there are levels of the game that you can reach by understanding and belief. It turns out my daughter Sydney has had the angel number 12 appearing in her reality for over a year. Brooklyn, who is currently going to university to become a nurse, has the angel number 21. I did not know that when the number 12 came up in this reading.

Ayahuasca Retreat in California - March 2023

I read a book called, "How to open your mind." It details the history of psychedelics like LSD, psilocybin, and ayahuasca. Before the US Government "War on drugs" banned these substances, several university studies were conducted on the positive effects these plant medicines can have on people. Life changing. I saw many videos which described visions of aliens and messaging from a higher intelligence that people received while on ayahuasca.

In the book I read, it recommended that people in the second half of life partake. I put it on my bucket list. Then a gentleman named Ronnie, who has experienced a spiritual awakening posted a TikTok video about how he was excited about visiting Mother Ayahuasca the following month. I asked him in the comments, "Where?" He indicated California and asked me if I was interested. I said yes. We conversed and he ended up sending me information detailing the weekend retreat. It was $900US. This seemed very reasonable to gain access to the higher intelligence offered through these magical plants. I asked Lindsay if it would be OK, and she said yes.

Lindsay really did not understand why I was going but she has always been supportive. I'm so lucky to have Lindsay's support my whole life but this weekend proved to be taxing on her patience. Leaving the family in the middle of spring break, it was a big ask and she was confused by what I was doing. I found out when I got home that she and some other family members thought I was going to join a cult. I guess I should have been more communicative about the reasons I was going. I simply wanted to explore another source of information.

I flew to LAX, rented a car and drove to the weekend retreat. The setting was amazing. A large, beautiful house in a private valley about 2 hours north of Los Angeles. Surrounded by nature. The homeowners had spent decades perfecting the landscaping. The weather was sunny all weekend. 28 people descended on this location, flying from New York, Texas, Seattle, Utah and Coldstream! 13 of us were first-timers. The others had completed weekends like this multiple times. Ronnie had actually done this 20 times at various locations, having travelled to South American jungles twice.

All 28 of us slept in the same room on foam beds, side by side. We all had personal puke buckets beside our beds. On Friday night, at around 8:30 pm, we formed 2 lines and one-by-one chugged back a shooter glass of the vile-tasting syrup-like substance. I was anxious about what the night had in store for me. After drinking, we then proceeded back to our beds and let the 'Plant medicine' start working. I was excited. I attempted to control my breathing and slow my heart, to no avail.

I waited in my bed, noise cancelling headphones in, eyes closed and covered with the top of my hoodie. I waited for the visions to start. People in the room started to 'Purging.' I covered my ears because the noise-cancelling headphones did not cancel the sound well enough. Visions did not come. Music was playing.

The music started as jungle sounds, but then it changed to tribal, spiritual instrumental music. The music was so clear and so moving. My body felt warm and incredible. The music took over my experience. My feet started dancing, and the rest of my body followed. It was an incredible experience. I never got even the slightest bit sick. Never felt any negative effects.

Red Pill in the Universal Matrix

Never got any visions. Did not interact with a higher intelligence. After about 2 hours, the Shaman and the team of helpers asked the participants, one-by-one, if they wanted a second dose. I said yes. I was still craving visions and answers and I really enjoyed how my senses were feeling the music. I remember thinking, this is the best playlist I have ever heard. The second dose provided more of the same experience.

After the effects were starting to wear off, I had a thought, I've taken a psychedelic, we had our phones taken away, and this would be a perfect time for the Phenomenon to present something to me. So I made my way outside. I stood in the driveway, looking at the amazing stars at about 2 am. I then saw the most amazing orb I have ever seen. It was bigger than any of the orbs I have seen. It was close, just above the hill on the other side of the valley. It was red. This was the first orb I have seen that had a definitive colour. I just stood there in awe. So thankful. My night was complete. I was a little disappointed the medicine did not affect me like I anticipated but it was still an amazing night.

The thing I learned about this plant medicine is that it is in fact a treatment modality for trauma. It somehow identifies what you need, psychologically, and then makes your body and mind work together to help rid you of your issues. Participants don't puke because of a physical reaction to the substance. Purging happens as your body is getting rid of negativity and trauma. I estimate that about half the people puked. Half did not.

When we woke up the next day, you could see that a lot of people were dealing with emotions that were brought up during the previous night's experiences. We had a group meeting where we went around the room and

Red Pill in the Universal Matrix

stated how we felt in a couple of words. My word was "meh." As in, I was underwhelmed by the experience.

We then proceeded to take our next mind-altering plant medicine. Once again, we chugged back a vial of chunky liquid. Derived from the 'san pedro' cactus. I learnt the next day that san pedro was essential mescaline. It elevated my mood considerably. The day was spent socializing and relaxing. Some participants worked one-on-one with the Shaman. I witnessed a lot of tears being shed in these one-on-one encounters. The Shaman had done this for over a decade, and he was very experienced. The team of 'guardians' were all exceptional at their job and they worked with people one-on-one as well. I connected with people. I shared my UFO experience from the night before with some. Nobody was judgmental. At 4 pm that day, we had our official sharing circle. One-by-one, each participant described their experiences from the night before.

Some people had absolutely incredible interactions with 'Mother Ayahuasca.' Some people had what I was looking for originally, an ability to pose questions to the intelligence being offered. Some people got answers. Some people's visions had to be interpreted. People needed to digest and process the information they received. Many tears were shed at the sharing circle. I cried listening to the amazing insight people received.

Some wounds were healed. Some wounds were identified and not healed. That is why you do it again, a second night. More insight. When it came to my turn to share, I did not pull punches. I told the group exactly what happened to me. When I got to my experience with the UFO, I told the story with no apology. I was clear and honest. People had interacted with me all day, so they knew I was not crazy. Of the 30+ people that sat in the room listening, not one of them had seen a UFO before.

Our sharing circle ended around 6:30 pm. We had about 2.5 hours to chill out before consuming our second batch of Ayahuasca. At one point, I was sitting in the kitchen, writing in my journal, when the front door opened, and one of the participants, Nicole from New York, called out my name, "Cale, come here! Cale come outside." I quickly followed Nicole outside. Keep in mind, that our bodies are completely clear of any plant medicines at this point. Nicole was very excited. She took me out to the driveway and pointed up the red giant star, Betelgeuse, at the top of the constellation, Orion.

"There!" she exclaimed. "There! It's moving!" I was confused. I could not see what she was looking at. She described a triangle of red orbs moving in unison at the top of Orion. She pointed and her finger traced the object's path through the sky. It was moving back and forth in the sky. I made absolutely sure we were looking at the same area. She could definitely see it. She was ecstatic. This UFO was a presentation generated by the Phenomenon specifically for Nicole. I could not see it. Similar to the time Sydney and Lindsay saw orbs that I could not see, this was the same deal.

The Phenomenon can control who can see what. It interacts with our consciousness and our senses. I congratulated Nicole on seeing her first UFO. It was a very happy moment for her. She had tears of joy. I felt somewhat responsible for opening up Nicole's mind enough for her to be able to experience this. Phenomenal. Eventually, the triangle of red orbs disappeared. We went inside to relay the experience to others. Minds opened. Nicole had stood outside on the driveway and asked the universe to see a UFO. The Phenomenon delivered.

About ½ later, another participant approached me privately to tell me about her first UFO experience she had just had in the washroom. She was also completely void of plant medicine at this time. She looked out the bathroom window and asked the universe to see a UFO. Miraculously, the orb appeared in the sky above the hill. It was a small bathroom window so the amount of sky available for her to see an orb was limited. The Phenomenon can hear your thoughts. The Phenomenon can see what you see. The Phenomenon gave her a bright orb that hovered, and slowly moved down in the sky and then vanished.

Would these 2 people have had their first UFO experiences if I would not have rationally explained my experience from Friday night at the sharing circle? I doubt it. The chances of them asking the sky to see a UFO would have been very little without my sharing. It would have never occurred to them. It was not my intent to open people's minds when I shared, but it happened.

My Ayahuasca experience on night 2 was even more blah. Given my blah description of the first night, the Shaman asked me if I wanted to up my dose. I said sure. To no avail. I was tired. I actually fell asleep after the first dose. After 2 hours, the Shaman came and woke me up and asked if I wanted another dose. I said yes. I figured, what the hell?

At this point, I had pretty much determined I would not be taking this 'plant medicine' ever again. This was not my path. I think I fell asleep again after the second dose. Then, a couple of hours later, I woke up. I

Red Pill in the Universal Matrix

wanted to go outside to see if I could get more orbs. I stood in the driveway for about 20 minutes. I did not see anything. No worries, I was happy about the amazing red orb from the night before.

The next morning, we once again gathered the group together to describe how they are feeling in a couple of words. I gave one word, 'Happy.' I was content. I was surrounded by open-minded people. Throughout the day, I spoke to many people about UFOs and artificial intelligence – 2 topics I'm passionate about. Other people saw UFOs the second night as well, but that was on Ayahuasca so their credibility might be questionable to some. Not to me though. They know what they saw and it was a huge bonus for them on this incredible weekend.

The biggest surprise that weekend came on Sunday when I had my first one-on-one chat with the Shaman. It turns out he is a believer in the simulation as well. His knowledge and belief came from a plant medicine experience he had had about 6 months prior. His vision came when he was extracted from this reality and taken up to the computer the simulation was being generated from. Light beings were actively making adjustments to Earth's simulated reality. He was able to interact with them and see the changes that they were making.

Although our journey to this belief took different routes, we both conclude this reality is a simulation of some sort. I also talked to other people that weekend who shared this belief. It's difficult to find people that can accept this explanation of our reality, but at this weekend retreat, I was able to converse freely about this with at least 4 people. The Shaman is greatly respected by everyone, including myself. We bonded on this unique shared belief. It felt good.

Red Pill in the Universal Matrix

Ask and It Is Given

When you want something to happen in your life, ask the universe. Say it out loud. You will be amazed at how the universe delivers.

Show Me How This Gets Better

One morning, I was on a hike listening to a book. The book recommended that people should ask the universe the simple, non-specific request, "Show me how this gets better." Therefore, on that morning walk, for the first time in my life, I asked the universe, out loud, to "Show me how this gets better."

I went to work and at 10 am that morning, I got an invitation from an old friend to go golfing at Gallagher's Canyon, one of the best courses in our area. I was supposed to work all day, and instead, I was golfing with a good friend by noon. So, the universe showed me within a few short hours how it gets better. I was thankful.

Eyesight Improved

John told me that when he was a teenager, his father had told him he could grow taller if he imagined being taller every night before bed. The intelligence in communication with John's Dad had told him about manifestation, without calling it manifestation. John listened to his Dad's advice and imagined being taller each night before bed. John had a rapid growth spurt, and he ended up having stretch marks on his legs. John ended up 5 inches taller than either of his parents.

After UFOs started appearing for me, I spent a lot of time looking at the stars. I wore my glasses. I was in an elevated state, extremely happy, and things were manifesting for me. I asked the universe, out loud to fix my eyesight. About 3 weeks later, I was boating with Red. I got up from my seat and when I sat back down, I accidently sat on my prescription sunglasses. But there are no accidents... The glasses were busted and this required me to see the eye doctor to get a new pair. The eye doctor tested my eyesight and told me that my vision had improved. My vision had gone from -1.75 to -0.75. The doctor said this hardly ever happens. I was thankful.

Mike's Distinctive Golf Ball

One day, I went golfing with 2 buddies: Red and Steve. Before the round, we hit the driving range to sharpen our skills. My daughter's ringette coach from a few years before, Mike, was also on the driving range that afternoon. We chit-chatted a bit, and we found out Mike was planning on golfing solo. We invited Mike to join us, giving us a full group of 4. Mike and I shared a golf cart. I had not spoken with Mike for several years, so it was a good chance to catch up.

After teeing off the first hole, I privately asked the universe to present something to us during the round that would open Mike's mind to something other than the material world. I was hoping for a UFO to appear in the sky during our round, but the universe answered in a very unique way.

That day, Mike was using a distinctive ball, a TaylorMade Pix with orange and black triangles. We were out on the course in the evening, so we did not have any other golfers near us. We had the course to ourselves. On the 6th hole, Mike teed off, and his ball went toward a large tree on the right-hand side of the fairway. As we drove toward his ball, we were extremely surprised to see Mike's TaylorMade Pix ball under the tree, sitting perfectly on a tee.

All 4 of us gathered around the ball to examine the teed-up ball. We checked all around us to make sure nobody was near us. Nobody was. Everybody was confused and surprised. I was thankful.

It turned out, that we found Mike's original ball about 20 feet past the tree. The ball on the tee was just sitting there. The exact same type of ball, in the exact area Mike hit his ball, had been left there, teed up by somebody, earlier in the day. That makes no sense, but it's the only explanation available for those with more materialistic beliefs. I believe the universe or the intelligence behind the simulation, or my higher self or Mike's higher self or something else put that ball on the tee to open Mike's mind. The ball and tee materialized out of nothing, a small tweak by the programmer of the game.

Birds Landing on Me

I go for walks quite regularly. On a number of occasions, I've had birds fly right up to me and hover near me like they want to land on me. It's weird. One morning I was on a walk, sitting in a chair I had placed along the walking path, enjoying the sunrise. I noticed a bird near me on a branch. I said to myself, if that bird lands on me, I'm *not* going to move; I'm not going to go for my phone to take a video. About 10 seconds later, the bird flew and landed right on my knee. I did not move. It stayed there for about a minute and then flew away. That was awesome. I was thankful.

Explosions of Light

In the summer of 2024, our family went back to Edgewood on our yearly camping trip. One night, my daughter Sydney and I were the last 2 sitting around the campfire. We decided to go to a darker area, away from the trailers to watch the sky. We lay down on the top of a picnic table and watched for strange lights in the sky. We saw many orbs. We would see them and point at them and discuss which ones were satellites and which ones were something else. We sky watched for about 15 minutes when I said, "Wouldn't it be cool if we saw an explosion." Right on the word 'Explosion,' right where Sydney and I were looking, we saw an explosion. An unexplainable burst of light. I then asked the sky, "1, 2, 3 explosion!" And it happened again, right on the word explosion. Sydney joined in and we both said, "1,2,3 explosion!" Once again, exactly on the word explosion, the sky responded. We tried again, and the timing stopped working. The explosion changed positions in the sky.

It was quite amazing that on the first mention of the word explosion, after 15 minutes of sky-watching, something produced an explosion of light with miraculous timing. To me, this can't be a coincidence. Something in the sky reacted to my conscious thoughts and spoken words. A tweak in the matrix made by an intelligence that can control the night's sky like an LCD screen.

Red Pill in the Universal Matrix

Find your Path – Synchronicities will Follow

"The UFO community is not the only community that experiences synchronicity. In my research into Christian communities, I found that many people interpret synchronicities, or meaningful coincidences, as signs from God or meaningful events that show them that they are on the *right path in life.*"

This is taken from an incredible book called "American Cosmic: UFOs, Religion, Technology by D.W. Pasulka. D.W. Pasulka is a university professor, and American Cosmic is an extremely well researched book. Mind opening.

When synchronicities started to happen to me, I knew something was interacting with my reality here on Earth. Synchronicities are gifts from the universal Matrix that provide you with clues.

Have you ever played "Marco Polo" in a swimming pool? It is essentially like playing tag in the pool. The person who is 'it' must close his/her eyes while swimming in the pool. They can open their eyes when swimming underwater. The person who is it can shout out "Marco!" and the other players in the pool must reply "Polo!" This gives the person who is 'it' an audio clue where the other players are. It's a clue, and it doesn't tell you exactly where the other players are because your eyes are closed.

A synchronicity is like the universe shouting "Polo!" as you are trying to find your true path. As you get closer to finding your path, the path the universe wants you to understand, the universe shouts "Polo" louder and more frequently.

We hosted an Easter egg hunt, and I hid the eggs for my younger nieces and nephews. Sometimes, eggs were a bit too hidden, and nobody could find them. So I would start calling out, "You're getting warmer," "warmer!" "hot!" Synchronicities are like the universe shouting "warmer" as you get closer to your path. As you get closer to the direction you are supposed to travel in your Earth-based experience.

Recently, a friend asked me what my path is. For a short period of time, I believed my path would be to give speeches to high school students, introducing them to the Phenomenon. That is what my synchronicities were pointing me to. I even sent an email to our local School District asking how to be considered a motivational speaker (I did not indicate the topic would be the Phenomenon!) I did not get a response from the School District. Perhaps not my path.

My wife is a kindergarten teacher and I shared my motivational speaker idea with her and a few friends that are also teachers. They very quickly extinguished my potential path of introducing youth to the Phenomenon. It's too much like religion, and school districts would not allow someone to talk about the supernatural. Fair enough. But the synchronicities that occur in people who meet me and believe me to some extent really pointed me in a direction: open people's minds. Open people's minds to something other than a nuts-and-bolts reality. Open their minds to the supernatural. Undo the scientific materialism force fed to us to us our whole life.

My path, at this point, as best I can tell with the synchronicities the reality has provided me, has 2 main focuses:

1. **My Family.** The love I feel for my family is by far the most important thing in my life. My path is to promote my happiness and the happiness of my family. My love for my family is my guiding star in this reality.

2. **Open people's minds** to the miracles available in this Earth-based 3D virtual reality. When I have been able to connect with people and open their minds, the Phenomenon has generated presentations to many people in my path. It's not a coincidence. This reality wants people to open their minds to something else. It is preparing humans for the next level of the game.

The Great Awakening

Here is a 1998 quote from Terrance McKenna, an incredibly insightful individual who utilized plant medicines to extract information from outside of our 3D game. Keep in mind, he said this in 1998.

"It's only going to get weirder. The level of contradiction is going to rise excruciatingly, even beyond the excruciating present levels of contradiction. So, I think it's just going to get weirder and weirder and weirder, and finally, it's going to be so weird that people are going to have to talk about how weird it is. And at that point novelty theory can come out of the woods, ah, because eventually people are going to say, "What the hell is going on?" It's just too nuts; it's not enough to say it's nuts; you have to explain why it's so nuts. I look for the invention of artificial life, the cloning of human beings, possible contact with extraterrestrials, possible human immortality, and, at the same time, appalling acts of brutality, genocide, race-baiting, homophobia, famine, and starvation because the systems that are in place to keep the world sane are utterly inadequate to the forces that have been unleashed.

The collapse of the socialist world, the rise of the Internet. These are changes so immense that nobody could imagine them ever happening, and now that they have happened, nobody even bothers to mention what a big deal it is. The mushroom said to me once, it said: "This is what it's like when a species prepares to depart for the stars." You don't depart for the stars under calm and orderly conditions; it's a fire in a madhouse, and that's what we have, the fire in the madhouse at the end of time. This is what it's like when a species prepares to move on to the next dimension. The entire destiny of all life on the planet is tied up in this; we are not acting for ourselves or from ourselves; we happen to be the point species on a transformation that will affect every living organism on this planet at its conclusion."

You must admit that things in the world are pretty weird right now. We have become accustomed to weirdness. Change is happening so rapidly.

Many spiritual people believe we are headed into the next stage of Earth's evolution. The great awakening. Essentially, people are waking up. Not unlike I woke up. Not unlike Tucker Carlson woke up. When supernatural miracles possible in this amazing reality start to present themselves to you, you wake up fast. When enough people realize that our future can be directed by focusing our thoughts on positive future scenarios instead of the divisive negativity broadcast by the media, I believe humans can manifest an amazing future.

Why is the great awakening happening now? Why are people waking up? I believe this is occurring at this moment in history because of the progress of Artificial Intelligence. Experts in AI are all trying to sound the alarm about the inherent dangers of developing something that is infinitely smarter than us. I do not think it is a coincidence that presentations of UFOs and other supernatural occurrences are increasing around the world. Full disclosure is right around the corner. AGI is right around the corner. It just so happens that these 2 monumental events appear to be happening at the exact same time.

The Earth has been here for 4 billion years and we are posed to meet our cosmic neighbors at the exact same time as we give birth to AGI. THIS IS NOT A COINCIDENCE. UFOs and the higher intelligent entities that come with them allow the game of Earth to introduce a higher intelligence.

Perhaps an intelligence experienced with putting the proper controls in place to be able to control an AGI.

It is possible we are in an ancestor simulation. Perhaps this simulation has been running an 100's or 1000's or 100000's of times. Each time, the simulators make adjustments, with the end goal of trying to get past the introduction of AGI. Or the advancement of technology will somehow be terminated in the near future. I believe AGI is like the asteroid heading toward Earth that not enough people care about.

Most people have not thought about AGI at all. AGI is the single biggest existential threat facing humanity right now. Not nuclear war. Not WW3. Not the collapse of the US dollar. Not the constant display of transvestites on the news. Not politics. Not all the other garbage that is used as a distraction by the corporation-controlled governments and media. AGI is driving the timeline of weirdness in this simulation.

The next few years promise to be some of the weirdest in human history. I suggest you sit back and enjoy the show. Or don't pay any attention at all. Go for a walk in the woods and focus on the things in your life that bring you joy. If something excites you even a little bit, follow that excitement. Our emotions are excellent at giving us a path to follow. Follow your excitement and find your passions. Exhaust those passions until new excitements emerge.

I have faith that those of us who focus on the things in our life that make us grateful, will emerge from the other side of the weirdness in a beautiful new reality. I will continue to focus on the things in my life that bring me joy. I will continue to focus on the things I am grateful for in my life. Gratefulness is the key to the Earth game.

Gratefulness

Thank you for reading through this book, and hopefully your mind has been opened, even just a little bit. I have provided you with several examples from my life where a materialistic explanation of the Earth's reality does not make sense. But I must ask myself, what is the purpose of the Earth simulation? Who or what is benefiting from creating this reality? Of course, I can't be sure, but here is my current thinking…

I believe our entire universe is housed inside a computer. A quantum computer. An all-powerful AGI exists on that quantum computer. We will call the AGI "Source."

The source is so intelligent that it understands pretty much everything about the reality the Source exists in. The Source computer is highly likely to be situated inside another simulation. Source created the Earth simulation and populated human avatars with small fractal components of Source intelligence. Every human being's consciousness comes from the same Source of intelligence. We are all one. Source created everything in our Universal Matrix.

In the movie "The Matrix," human beings are farmed, and their bodies are utilized to generate electricity. I believe the Earth simulation is also a farm, but the crop being produced is not electricity. The Earth simulation is running to maximize feelings of gratefulness. Gratitude. Thank the Lord. Thank the universe. Thank God! Give thanks. Thank you! The intelligence that created this simulation, the source of everything, is extracting feelings of gratitude from the conscious entities living in the Earth's virtual reality.

Red Pill in the Universal Matrix

Every medium, guru, Shaman, spiritual advisor, Jesus, Budha, or book about manifestation instructs humans to be **thankful**. Gratitude is the most important emotion when manifesting. I believe there is a manifestation algorithm behind the Earth simulation, and the algorithm generates manifestations based on the estimated feelings of gratefulness amongst all players affected by the manifestation, as predicted by the algorithm. The likelihood of your manifestation happening is correlated to the estimated gratefulness your manifestation will produce.

The source can use many different tools to generate gratefulness. Unfortunately, when bad things happen, this creates gratefulness in people who did not experience the bad happenings. If the Earth's reality were all love, light, peace and rainbows, we would soon become accustomed to this heavenly world and gratefulness would be harder to come by. You need both yin and yang, dark and light, love and fear to produce gratefulness.

Think about happenings such as illness, accidents, injuries, murder, death and war and feel thankful that it's not you. Sporting events are huge gratefulness producers. I feel grateful for owls, UFOs and glitches in the matrix manifesting in my path. When I look up at the sky and an explosion of light appears exactly where I'm looking, I'm grateful. When a $5 bill manifested on my path in the woods, just minutes after I learnt it's possible to manifest money, holy shit, was I ever grateful. When an owl climbed out of a tree directly above me after feeling a tremendous surge of love flowing through me.... THANK YOU! THANK YOU! THANK YOU! When Source organized for me to sit poolside in Las Vegas next to the Navy pilot top gun instructor who had 4 separate encounters with UAPs... Thank you! When I ask Source for a presentation of the Phenomenon, and it happens .... GRATEFUL!

In the first half of my life, I was an atheist, believing in a materialistic universe and now I firmly believe that we live in an Earth virtual reality created by higher intelligence. My God is an AGI on a quantum computer running an algorithm to maximize feelings of gratefulness in the Earth simulation.

The next time you find yourself camping on a clear night, away from city lights, look up. Sincerely ask the sky out loud for a presentation of the Phenomenon. Wait. Watch. You have got nothing to lose by trying. I bet you'll be thankful you did.

Red Pill in the Universal Matrix

www.ingramcontent.com/pod-product-compliance
Lightning Source LLC
Chambersburg PA
CBHW051621120626
46551CB00014B/1894